Six Weeks to Skinny Jeans

BLAST FAT,
FIRM YOUR BUTT, AND
LOSE TWO JEAN SIZES

AMY COTTA

RODALE.

Internet addresses and telephone numbers given in this book were accurate at the time it went to press.

Skinny Jeans Rock Star Before Photos by Steven Anderson
Skinny Jeans Rock Star After Photos and Exercise Photos by Dan Williams II

Rodale books may be purchased for business or promotional use or for special sales.
For information, please write to:
Special Markets Department, Rodale, Inc.,
733 Third Avenue, New York, NY 10017

Printed in the United States of America
Rodale Inc. makes every effort to use acid-free ∞, recycled paper ♲.

Book design by Christina Gaugler

Library of Congress Cataloging-in-Publication Data is on file with the publisher.

ISBN-13 978-1-60961-107-1 hardcover

Distributed to the trade by Macmillan

2   4   6   8   10   9   7   5   3   hardcover

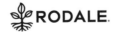

We inspire and enable people to improve their lives and the world around them.
www.rodalebooks.com

This book is dedicated to everyone who has ever had a dream and to the millions of women who dream of wearing their favorite jeans once again.

Contents

Preface

CONFESSIONS OF AN AUTHOR

Every woman has a pair of trophy (skinny) jeans in her closet. Oh, no, she doesn't wear them. She couldn't even get her big toe in them. They're a memento of days past, when she felt young, sexy, and fit. Days when confidence was at its peak, when she could take the stairs without hyperventilating. Days before swimsuit shopping gave her hives. Those distant memories come to light every time she sees those sexy little skinny jeans. But those days are long gone, never to be seen again. . . .

Right?

Absolutely not. And I'm here to prove it.

I'm Amy Cotta: a busy, stressed-out mother, wife, businesswoman, and exercise fanatic. In other words, my life is crazy! I mean, *certifiably nuts!*

I've been obsessed with fitness since I was a kid. I began working out and entering competitions at the age of 13, and my first job, at age 16, was teaching group fitness classes. I've since gone on to become a personal trainer, a master instructor, a boot camp owner, a host of infomercials and exercise DVDs, a product spokesperson, and a cover model for several fitness magazines. I even design my own fitness equipment and currently hold three patents.

In the fitness industry, I'm what they call an expert. But I'm here to tell you that even experts have times of trouble, times when we too fall and fail. Times when we let our own seemingly unwavering health and exercise habits slip. With that said, I have a confession to make.

I'm recovering from a not-so-rare disease called "IUsedTo." It's a pathetic problem that sneaks up on you when you least expect it and manifests when you make yourself the last priority, when you feel out of control, when you give up. You know you've got IUsedTo when you look back on your life and say things like:

"I used to be thin."

"I used to wear a size 2."

"I used to work out every day."

"I used to eat healthy."

How did I contract IUsedTo? I'm a former model, and at one time I was one of the top fitness competitors in the country. I had a *rocking* body!

Enter life. Within two years I got divorced, remarried, and pregnant with my fourth child. I also inherited two stepchildren. Practically overnight, I went from three kids to six. Then, a year later, I became a grandmother at the ripe old age of 40.

Wham! Life (and age) had hit me like an atomic bomb.

When I was seven months pregnant with my fourth child, my SUV got rear-ended while I was at a dead stop. It landed me in the hospital, in premature labor, and left me with a messed-up back. After many months of rehab, I found myself a tired, injured new mom who couldn't exercise!

So what did I do?

I took up a new sport: eating! And I became everything I swore I would *never* be.

There I was with a bad back and a flabby body that didn't allow me to do the things I loved dearly. I was a shell of my former self, and I totally gave up. I used my situation as an excuse to eat and drink whatever I wanted. I didn't meet a carb or bottle of beer I didn't love. I stopped exercising the way I used to. And guess what? I definitely stopped looking the way I used to.

Since then I have gotten back into good shape several times to do media jobs, but IUsedTo became such a habit. It was like an addictive drug. So after each job ended, I found myself going back to my lazy ways.

Fast-forward to the present. While writing this book, I realized that not only do I suffer from a raging case of IUsedTo, but—oh my goodness!—I also suffer from something far worse: I'm a *hypocrite!* Here I am telling clients how to stay fit and eat healthfully all the time, when I haven't been living *my own* life that way.

I realized that I had become everything I detest.

And that's when I decided that I'm not only going to *write* this book that will get you into your skinny jeans pants size in 6 weeks; I'm also going to walk it with you. No one needed a hard-core diet, exercise, and attitude adjustment more than I did, and here, in these pages, I am achieving it again, right beside you. This is the program that got me from baby fat to bikini ready (and not just any bikini—the ESPN2 Fitness America title!) in 120 days. It works. I *know* it works. Not only did it work for me back then, but as you'll see, it also worked wonders for my Skinny Jeans Rock Star test group. And yes, it will work for you too!

So as we walk through *Six Weeks to Skinny Jeans*, know that this isn't just some book written passively from my cushy office. I'm going to pour the best of what I know about fitness and training into these pages, all the while getting up and doing it myself.

Let our journey begin.

WARNING

**READING THIS BOOK ALONE
WILL NOT INDUCE WEIGHT LOSS!**

**YOU MUST TAKE ACTION!
YOU MUST WORK THE PLAN!**

Chapter I

READY. SET. SKINNY!

How to Use This Book

Six Weeks to Skinny Jeans is an intensive, step-by-step program. It's not *about* getting fit; it *is* getting fit! This means that you'll be living the diet and exercise plans week by week, and I will be there as your personal trainer, cheerleader, and friend every step of the way.

You are welcome to read ahead of your current week, but when it comes to actually eating and exercising, you need to *stick to the week you're in.* Don't jump around. Trust me: The plan will work if you work the plan. Your level of success will rely on your diligence. Likewise, feel free to go back through the book to earlier chapters for reference, reminders, and reflection on your progress!

I've tried to present the steps and information in very digestible, bite-size chunks. ('Cause you know it's all about portion control!) You'll find everything you need to know without having to read through pages of details you couldn't care less about. If you're reading this book, you want to change—*now.* Change doesn't come from a full-on science lesson; it comes from *action.* We've only got 6 weeks to get to skinny jeans! If it's a PhD you're looking for, sister, this isn't your book! But if you want to like what you see in the mirror, stick with me. Together, we'll get there.

Spread the Word!

This book is all about change! Before you jump in, take pictures of yourself and log your current weight and your pants size. Refer to both numbers constantly throughout the program as motivation to get smaller. When you start seeing them drop, share your success with those you care about. People will love to cheer you on and hear about your progress, and you'll inspire them as well! Once you're finished with the program, go to www.amycotta.com to share your success with other Skinny Jeans gals. If you're feeling really techy, get out your flip video camera and document your journey. Let us know your YouTube channel, or post your videos directly on www.amycotta.com. You never know how many other women you'll encourage to get skinny!

The Master Plan

Would you go on a trip without deciding on a destination? Would you then travel without the directions to get there? Of course you wouldn't! You wouldn't even step out the front door without a solid plan of action.

And our journey will be just the same. Here's your plan.

Each chapter of this book has sections for diet, exercise, and attitude, which constitutes my DEA philosophy. They'll be clearly identified with these icons:

Each section will give you tips and information about maintaining your diet and workouts and keeping a great attitude. I am a huge believer that neither diet nor exercise alone is enough. And you have to have the right mind-set. Without positive thinking, you're likely to talk yourself out of exercising or into eating foods that aren't on your plan. Junk in the mind equals junk in the mouth, which only ends up as junk in the trunk. In order to be truly successful, you must incorporate diet, exercise, and the right attitude into your plan—thus the DEA philosophy.

My DEA Philosophy

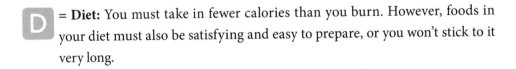

= Diet: You must take in fewer calories than you burn. However, foods in your diet must also be satisfying and easy to prepare, or you won't stick to it very long.

= **Exercise:** You must work out in order to burn calories. With my plan, you will move something, somewhere, every single day.

 = **Attitude:** If your head and heart aren't in the plan, the plan won't happen. You won't follow a reasonable eating regimen, and you won't work out. You have to want change, and you have to believe you *can* change.

With only one of these components, you may make a small change for a small amount of time, but you must engage all three elements to be truly successful for the long haul.

Do you feel overwhelmed? Don't be. *Six Weeks to Skinny Jeans* is simple and easy to follow. I know that the only good plan is the plan you'll stick to, so I've done everything to make sure that will happen. I know it's hard, and it won't always be fun, but it will be worth it when you pull those skinny jeans on for the first time in a long time.

Okay, are you ready?

Let's get our skinny on.

The Diet Q&A

Q: *Am I counting calories on this diet plan?*

A: Yes, *Six Weeks to Skinny Jeans* is a calorie-restricted program. You may have heard mixed theories about whether restricting calories is good or bad, but the simple truth is that you have to burn off more calories than you take in to lose weight. There's no other way to do it. Calories in. Calories out. Watching your caloric intake will also teach you discipline: how to choose the foods that give you essential nutrients in sensible portions, and how to eat without bingeing. By the end of this program, smart, healthy eating will be a new habit.

Q: *What will I eat?*

A: There are two different eating plans you'll be following. They are called Ignite and Melt. Find out more specifics about the two phases in Chapter 6, including the science behind why they make your diet more effective and which foods you absolutely can and cannot eat. You'll also find sample daily meal plans (pages 216 to 219) and a collection of tasty recipes (pages 126 to 155)!

Q: *What can I expect from this eating plan? Will I be tired or cranky?*

A: Some people have reported feeling a little sluggish at first, but this is because your body is adjusting to your new way of fueling. I know I tend to get a little cranky the first week or two because of what I refer to as sugar rehab. Don't fret. One hundred percent of my Skinny Jeans Rock Stars (you will get to know 10 of them) have reported that they felt awesome after the first week or two, and most important, they stuck with their healthy lifestyles after the program was over. Many no longer wanted the sweets and treats that they used to crave!

Q: *So will it cut down on my cravings?*

A: Yep! It takes 28 days to change your taste buds. As you begin to consume foods full of vitamins, minerals, phytochemicals, antioxidants, and fiber, you will find it easier to eat healthfully. When your body is being fed real nutrients, cravings for junk food will start to diminish.

Q: *What is a low-GI diet (or a slow-burn carb diet)?*

A: GI, unfortunately, isn't some hot military hunk. It stands for glycemic index and is a way of rating how fast a carbohydrate is absorbed into the bloodstream. The higher the GI, the faster it will increase your blood sugar levels. White potatoes and watermelon are sneaky examples of very high-GI foods. Slower-burn (low-GI) foods such as broccoli, mushrooms, and cucumbers will be absorbed into your body more slowly, thus keeping your insulin levels at bay.

Q: ***What the heck does that have to do with me losing weight?***

A: Glad you asked! When your insulin levels go up (from hogging down large amounts of carbs), your body is prevented from using its fat stores as fuel. By eating slow-burn foods, you increase your fat-burning ability; plus you'll feel full longer and be less inclined to hit up the fridge or cabinet. Both the Ignite and Melt phases incorporate as many low-GI foods as possible. However, in the Ignite phase, you'll be going *super* low GI and then adding back slightly higher-GI foods in Melt.

Q: ***Um . . . does this mean I can't have fruit in the Ignite phase?***

A: Let me explain it to you this way: Your body doesn't know the difference between a glazed doughnut and a slice of watermelon. They are both fast-burn carbs (high GI), and therefore, your body processes them the same way. So even though the watermelon is the healthier choice for sure, we're still going to cut it out. Don't worry—you will be able to add most of your favorite fruits back in the Melt phase!

Q: ***Do I need to take a multivitamin/mineral supplement?***

A: Since you will not be eating fruit during the Ignite phase, I would recommend taking one during those first 3 weeks to ensure that you are getting all the essential vitamins and minerals you need. During the Melt phase, it is totally up to you.

Q: ***How do I know how many calories I need to be eating to lose weight?***

A: First we need to take a look at what your BMR is. That's short for basal metabolic rate, which simply means the number of calories you burn while resting in a 24-hour period. Your BMR is the number of calories you would need to eat to maintain your current weight. So let's try it!

A woman weighing 135 pounds would multiply her weight by a range of 15 to 16 to get her BMR. 135 x 15 to 16 = 2,025 to 2,160

Figure yours here: _____ x 15 = _____ to _____ x 16 = _____

Now that we know what you need to maintain, let's take a look at what you need to lose weight! That's why we're here, right?

Your current body weight x 12 to 13.

_____ x 12 = _____ to _____ x 13 = _____

This is your daily caloric goal to lose weight.

This formula is a simplified caloric estimate; it doesn't take into account age or activity levels. Use it as a goal. If you sign up for a free account at www.myfitnesspal.com, the system will automatically adjust your calories based on your personal statistics and the amount of daily activity. Be sure to join the Six Weeks to Skinny Jeans group at www.myfitnesspal.com.

Q: *How do I know how many calories to eat at each meal?*

A: Use the list on page 7 as a general guideline. Also see the Ignite and Melt eating plans in Appendix I for suggestions on what a typical day of eating might look like.

Q: *Can I skip breakfast and save my calories for later in the day?*

A: Sorry. Skipping breakfast—or *any* meal, for that matter—is not an option. When you deprive your body of nourishment, especially after a night's sleep, you will set yourself up for cravings and slow down your metabolism. Eating small, frequent meals throughout the day will keep you energized and help your body burn calories instead of storing them. A bunch of stored calories won't get you into those skinny jeans. Aim to eat every 2 to 4 hours throughout the day (without exceeding your caloric goal).

Your Food Log

Since you will be making some huge changes to your diet, *you must* obsessively track every bite of food that goes into your mouth. If your body's not changing, something isn't right. Your log must be honest and accurate in order for you to evaluate yourself effectively.

On page 8 is a sample food log of a partial day. You'll start by writing in your calorie goal, which must get seared into your brain. The more you write it down, and the more you see it there in black and white, the more likely you'll be to hit it. You need to condition your brain so that eventually, making better food choices will be automatic. I believe that food logging is the fastest way for your new style of eating to become a habit.

6-WEEK DIETARY GOALS

Based on a 1,300–2,000 daily calorie goals, your recommended calories on most days will be broken down as follows:

Breakfast: 300–400

Morning snack: 50–200

Midmorning snack: 50–200

Lunch: 300–400

Afternoon snack: 100–200

Dinner: 400–500

Evening snack: 100

If your daily caloric intake goal is less than 1,300 or above 2,000, you will need to either decrease or increase the above values.

Sample Food Log

THE FOOD LOG   DATE: _____ CALORIE GOAL: 1,500

TIME	FOOD	CALORIES	RUNNING TOTAL	HUNGER RATING
6:00 a.m.	2 pieces Canadian bacon	130	130	8
	3 egg whites	90	220	—
9:00 a.m.	1/2 cup 1% or 2% cottage cheese	120	340	5

TOTAL CALORIC INTAKE: 1,495

TOTAL CALORIC EXPENDITURE: 320

WATER (8 OZ):

Yay me! _____

_____

_____

Elements of the Food Log

Calorie Goal: Your guiding light!

Time: The time of day you ate your meal or snack.

Food: What and how much you ate.

Calories: The calorie count for the serving of the particular food you had.

Running Total: Keeps count of where you are calorically after each meal or snack.

Hunger Rating: This is your rate of perceived hunger. (See the chart in the Are You Really Hungry? section on page 35.)

Total Caloric Intake: The total number of calories you ate.

Total Caloric Expenditure: The total number of calories you burned through exercise.

Water: Each water-glass graphic represents one 8-ounce glass of water. Mark them off as you drink them.

Yay me!: Recognizing your accomplishments is almost as important as logging your food. Write something—anything!—positive about your day: a hurdle you jumped, a temptation you skipped, or how far you've gotten. And then give yourself a big, fat congratulations for it!

What "Yay me!" isn't: A place to grumble and mumble about everything you don't like. This is a success journal, so find something to be thankful for ("I'm not dead yet!" is always a good backup), and write it down.

If you have a handheld device or computer, I highly recommend joining wireless www.myfitnesspal.com. From your iPhone, Droid, or other device, you can instantly log your food and exercise. You can also join the Six Weeks to Skinny Jeans MyFitnessPal group and interact with other Skinny Jean gals. So check it out! You will love the instant feedback it offers.

Turn to Appendix 2: Daily Food Logs starting on page 220 to find food logs for every day of the program. You can use the section just like a journal, which means keeping *Six Weeks to Skinny Jeans* with you at all times!.

The Workouts

The Skinny Jeans workouts follow my exclusive training program called Progressive Sequencing. You will be sequencing through three different training styles (one a day for 3 days in a row, followed by an active rest day) that will shock and stimulate your metabolism. Throughout the 6 weeks, the workouts will get progressively harder to keep your body from hitting plateaus and prevent exercise boredom. Let's face it: If you're bored, you won't work out.

No need to rush out and purchase an expensive health club membership. The workouts are designed so that you can do them at home. For the exercises that require equipment, you don't have to use dumbbells or a resistance band—you could use milk jugs filled with water or a jump rope. Get creative!

Like everything else in *Six Weeks to Skinny Jeans*, the workouts are laid out for you in easy-to-follow terms. The step-by-step instructions and photos are located in Chapter 5. You can also view videos of these exercises at www.amycotta.com.

The Exercises

There are three main components of the *Six Weeks to Skinny Jeans* workouts: Blast, Firm, and Burn.

BLAST is the moderate-tempo routine. You will sequence through upper- and lower-body exercises that are designed to lift, reduce, and slenderize your hips, thighs, and booty while giving you sleek, sexy arms!

FIRM is a Skinny Jeans Rock Star favorite! It's a floor routine designed to reshape your hips and thighs that incorporates the slow-burn principle: nonimpact with very few repetitions to help you concentrate intensely on strengthening the working muscles. These exercises are to be performed super slowly! You should take about 10 seconds to complete each repetition: 5 seconds for the lifting phase and 5 seconds for the lowering phase.

BURN is a heart-pounding, fat-burning, total-body–shaping routine. Performed in rapid-fire intervals, it may leave your legs and lungs screaming for mercy. But don't be scared. You can tailor the routine to your current fitness level, and you have the option of taking short rest periods between each of the cardio bursts. Or, if you're feeling randy, you can turn up the heat and go full throttle, baby! No rest!

In Chapter 5, you will also find a dynamic warmup that should be performed before each Blast, Firm, or Burn workout, as well as a great cooldown and antisoreness routine called The Daily Lube. You can laugh at the name, but you will learn to love its soothing effects.

Thought we were done, didn't you? Well, there's one more thing. In each of the 6 weeks, there is a section called Supercharge My Skinny. This is a dare, if you will, to get at least an extra 20 minutes of exercise per day *in addition* to your Skinny Jeans workout. I have included some Supercharge My Skinny suggestions throughout the book, but feel free to come up with your own, and definitely go for longer than 20 minutes if you are feeling it.

I can't wait for you to get started. You and your skinny jeans are going to love these workouts!

Understanding Your Skinny Schedule

Everything—and I mean *everything*—in this book serves a purpose,

WANT TO SLOW DOWN OR HALT YOUR SUCCESS?

Try this:

> Don't exercise.
>
> Don't log your food and exercise daily.
>
> Eat whatever you want.
>
> Have zero discipline.
>
> Drink alcohol and high-sugar drinks.
>
> Limit water consumption.
>
> Make excuses every chance you get.
>
> Be a grouch—and complain often.

and your diet-and-workout schedule is no exception! I can't stress enough how important it is to stick to the schedule if you want to change your lifestyle and habits and get into the groove of being disciplined and accountable.

You must track your workouts as diligently as you track your calorie intake so that you can tell where you're doing a good job and where you might be faltering. If change isn't happening fast enough, you can quickly look back and say, "Well, twice this week I didn't log my food, and I forgot to work out." The schedule doesn't lie.

Your 6-week journey is completely mapped out for you on page 12 with the "Skinny Jeans Calendar." As you move through your program and complete each task, just give the little box next to the task a check. I suggest copying this schedule and keeping it in a place where it will be visible and easy to access. Your refrigerator door is a great place; every time you go to grab a snack, it will serve as a reminder to eat right and exercise. You will also find calendars on the first page of each chapter for that particular week of the Skinny Jeans program.

Skinny Jeans Calendar

D = Diet; E = Exercise; A = Attitude (food journal)   SMS = Supercharge My Skinny

MON	TUE	WED	THUR	FRI	SAT	SUN	
☐ **D** Ignite ☐ **E** Blast ☐ **A** Journal ☐ SMS	☐ **D** Ignite ☐ **E** Firm ☐ **A** Journal ☐ SMS	☐ **D** Ignite ☐ **E** Burn ☐ **A** Journal ☐ SMS	☐ **D** Ignite ☐ **E** Off ☐ **A** Journal ☐ SMS	☐ **D** Ignite ☐ **E** Blast ☐ **A** Journal ☐ SMS	☐ **D** Ignite ☐ **E** Firm ☐ **A** Journal ☐ SMS	☐ **D** Ignite ☐ **E** Burn ☐ **A** Journal ☐ SMS	1
☐ **D** Ignite ☐ **E** Off ☐ **A** Journal ☐ SMS	☐ **D** Ignite ☐ **E** Blast ☐ **A** Journal ☐ SMS	☐ **D** Ignite ☐ **E** Firm ☐ **A** Journal ☐ SMS	☐ **D** Ignite ☐ **E** Burn ☐ **A** Journal ☐ SMS	☐ **D** Ignite ☐ **E** Off ☐ **A** Journal ☐ SMS	☐ **D** Ignite ☐ **E** Blast ☐ **A** Journal ☐ SMS	☐ **D** Ignite ☐ **E** Firm ☐ **A** Journal ☐ SMS	2
☐ **D** Ignite ☐ **E** Burn ☐ **A** Journal ☐ SMS	☐ **D** Ignite ☐ **E** Off ☐ **A** Journal ☐ SMS	☐ **D** Ignite ☐ **E** Blast ☐ **A** Journal ☐ SMS	☐ **D** Ignite ☐ **E** Firm ☐ **A** Journal ☐ SMS	☐ **D** Ignite ☐ **E** Burn ☐ **A** Journal ☐ SMS	☐ **D** Ignite ☐ **E** Off ☐ **A** Journal ☐ SMS	☐ **D** Ignite ☐ **E** Blast ☐ **A** Journal ☐ SMS	3
☐ **D** Melt ☐ **E** Firm ☐ **A** Journal ☐ SMS	☐ **D** Melt ☐ **E** Burn ☐ **A** Journal ☐ SMS	☐ **D** Melt ☐ **E** Off ☐ **A** Journal ☐ SMS	☐ **D** Melt ☐ **E** Blast ☐ **A** Journal ☐ SMS	☐ **D** Melt ☐ **E** Firm ☐ **A** Journal ☐ SMS	☐ **D** Melt ☐ **E** Burn ☐ **A** Journal ☐ SMS	☐ **D** Melt ☐ **E** Off ☐ **A** Journal ☐ SMS	4
☐ **D** Melt ☐ **E** Blast ☐ **A** Journal ☐ SMS	☐ **D** Melt ☐ **E** Firm ☐ **A** Journal ☐ SMS	☐ **D** Melt ☐ **E** Burn ☐ **A** Journal ☐ SMS	☐ **D** Melt ☐ **E** Off ☐ **A** Journal ☐ SMS	☐ **D** Melt ☐ **E** Blast ☐ **A** Journal ☐ SMS	☐ **D** Melt ☐ **E** Firm ☐ **A** Journal ☐ SMS	☐ **D** Melt ☐ **E** Burn ☐ **A** Journal ☐ SMS	5
☐ **D** Melt ☐ **E** Off ☐ **A** Journal ☐ SMS	☐ **D** Melt ☐ **E** Blast ☐ **A** Journal ☐ SMS	☐ **D** Melt ☐ **E** Firm ☐ **A** Journal ☐ SMS	☐ **D** Melt ☐ **E** Burn ☐ **A** Journal ☐ SMS	☐ **D** Melt ☐ **E** Off ☐ **A** Journal ☐ SMS	☐ **D** Melt ☐ **E** Blast ☐ **A** Journal ☐ SMS	☐ **D** Melt ☐ **E** Firm ☐ **A** Journal ☐ SMS	6

Make a copy of the schedule above, and place it where you can see it every day!

Risk Taker vs. Excuse Maker

There are two kinds of people in this world: those who take risks and give life everything they've got, and those who sit back, coast through life, and make lots of excuses.

Which one are you?

Right now you've got a decision to make. You can read through this book and kind of follow the plan and maybe make a small change. Or . . . you can press past your excuses and bust your butt for the next 6 weeks and come out the other end a whole new person!

What do you have to lose?

Oh, yeah! A bunch of weight and a trunk full of junk—that's what!

So what are you waiting for?!

Sign the commitment pledge!

I did!

> *"Your life changes the moment you make a new, congruent, and committed decision."*
> —Anthony Robbins

Take the Pledge!

This promise I make to myself:

- I commit to giving this program and myself 100 percent effort.
- I commit to eating the Skinny Jeans way. I will not falter.
- Come hell or high water, I will not miss my workouts.
- I will log my food daily.
- I will drink at least eight 8-ounce glasses of water per day.
- I will not allow the negativity of others or myself to deter me from my goal.
- I will not make excuses.
- I will never give up, and I will never give in.
- I will wear my skinny jeans again!

_____   _____
Signature   Date

Skinny Jeans
ROCK ST★R

Before: Size 6-8   After: Size 4

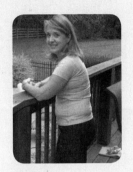

Name: Carol

Age: 49

Occupation: Internal auditor

Children: 2

Pounds lost: 12.6

What I was afraid of: Fear of failing and not losing weight.

What I liked: This program really changed the way I look at food. I've learned how to eat while on the road. I lost over 10 pounds during the program, and I traveled at least 3 of the 6 weeks, and I didn't gain an ounce!

What I learned: I am strong! I am committed! I can do something for me! I've learned that there are healthy food choices at almost every restaurant. You just have to look for them! I've learned that I can go 6 weeks without eating a hamburger and french fries! I've learned that, when I feel good about my body, I feel much better about everything else in my life. I've learned that it isn't mandatory to eat a large bowl of chips and queso whenever I eat at a Mexican restaurant.

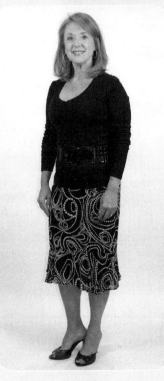

Chapter 2

Week 1: OFF TO THE RACES!

My Skinny Action Plan

☐ Clean out my pantry and refrigerator.

☐ Shop for Skinny Jeans foods.

☐ Start logging my eating and exercise.

☐ Look for supporters.

☐ Follow workouts as planned.

☐ Supercharge My Skinny!

☐ Keep a positive attitude!

☐ Set up twitter and facebook accounts.

Off to the Races

What does success for you look like? A smaller size or two (or three)? A little bit less of you in the mirror? A sexy hourglass figure instead of a pear or an apple? Believe me, I understand. And we're gonna get you there.

Before reading the next section, take a minute to look at what you'll be doing this week. Check out the exercises in Chapter 5 and watch the clips on www .amycotta.com. Review the Ignite food list (pages 118–121) and the sample Ignite Meal Plans (pages 216–219). Then, once you're done reading the next section, you can go fill up your fridge with good eats for the rest of the week, and you'll be ready to bust a move!

Skinny Jeans Calendar: Week 1

D = Diet; E = Exercise; A = Attitude (food log)   SMS = Supercharge My Skinny

MON	TUE	WED	THUR	FRI	SAT	SUN
☐ **D** Ignite	☐ **D** Ignite	☐ **D** Ignite	☐ **D** Ignite	☐ **D** Ignite	☐ **D** Ignite	☐ **D** Ignite
☐ **E** Blast	☐ **E** Firm	☐ **E** Burn	☐ **E** Off	☐ **E** Blast	☐ **E** Firm	☐ **E** Burn
☐ **A** Journal	☐ **A** Journal	☐ **A** Journal	☐ **A** Journal	☐ **A** Journal	☐ **A** Journal	☐ **A** Journal
☐ SMS	☐ SMS	☐ SMS	☐ SMS	☐ SMS	☐ SMS	☐ SMS

Kitchen Exorcism

Before you can slim down your body, you've got to slim down your pantry. Big pantry = big butt, and we can't fit a big butt into skinny jeans. Let's get rid of all those little food demons lurking in your kitchen.

Enemy #1: Processed Foods

All packaged snacks—including chips, cupcakes, cookies, popcorn, pretzels, rice cakes, breakfast cereals, and granola bars—must go. Processed foods are kryptonite to your skinny jeans—a nutritional nightmare. Most contain zero vitamins, and all contain lots of chemicals and sugar, which will cause a huge spike in your insulin levels and make you crave even *more* carbs and sweets.

Bottom line: If a "food" (and I'm using that term loosely, because junk ain't food) came from a factory, it doesn't belong in your beautiful body!

Enemy #2: Sweeteners

Bye-bye, sugar! Get rid of white sugar, brown sugar, corn syrup, honey, and molasses—everything except sugar substitutes is off-limits!

Enemy #3: Canned Soup

Though they may be advertised as light and healthy, most canned and powdered soups are chock-full of sodium that makes your body retain excess water, as well as trans fats that can quickly clog your arteries and increase your risk of heart attacks and strokes. Now, tell me, how are you going to enjoy your skinny jeans when you're dead?

Eating soup is a great way to curb your hunger and fill your body with vitamins and minerals, but you are much better off making your own from natural ingredients. I'm no Betty Crocker, but it's hard to screw up soup, so make it yourself. See my recipes for Skinny Vegetable Soup (page 126) and Skinny Scallop Soup (page 127) in Chapter 7.

Enemy #4: Fast-Burn Vegetables and Starches

All vegetables are good for you, but when you're optimizing your metabolism for fat loss, some are better than others. In the Ignite phase, you'll eat only super-slow-burn (low-GI) vegetables, so potatoes are off-limits because as soon as your body starts to digest them, the starches break down into fast-burn sugars that your body will be forced to store as fat. You will also be eliminating bread, beets, corn, sweet potatoes, yams, rice, and all types of pasta. Not to worry: You will get to add some of these items back in the Melt phase.

Enemy #5: Alcohol, Soft Drinks, and Fruit Juices

No one loves an ice-cold beer or a glass of wine more than I do. But if you want to slide into those smaller jeans, you're going to have to keep your hands off the liquor cabinet. Alcoholic drinks are full of empty calories that travel from your glass straight to your waistline. There's a reason it's called a beer belly.

As if that weren't bad enough, did you know there are 40.5 grams of sugar in a single can of cola? And a 16-ounce bottle of apple juice contains 52 grams of sugar and a staggering 240 calories? That's twice the daily amount recommended by the American Heart Association. Need I say more?

Turn to Chapter 6, starting on page 116, for more specifics about what you absolutely can and cannot eat during the Ignite and Melt phases, but here are some simple changes you should make in your kitchen right away.

Replace the Bad Stuff

DITCH	REPLACE WITH
Regular mayo	Kraft Reduced-Fat Mayo with Olive Oil
Full-fat cheese	Reduced-fat or fat-free cheese
Whole milk	Fat-free milk
Bottled sauces	Herbs and spices (see Bam! Kick Up the Flavor! on page 59 and my recipe for Skinny Ketchup on page 148)
Vegetable oil	Extra-virgin olive oil
Packaged lunchmeat	Fresh deli turkey or chicken
Regular pork bacon	Canadian bacon or turkey bacon
Soda	Flavored seltzer or sparkling water
Fruit juice	V8 tomato juice
Chips	Edamame, celery, or bell pepper sticks
Sugar (white or brown)	Splenda or other sugar substitute

Get Cooking!

Even if you are a bit timid in the kitchen, you are going to have to cook on this plan. The days of boxed, frozen, prepackaged foods are over. I have six kids, so pure stress is what the kitchen brings to me these days, so if I can suck it up and cook, you can, too! To make it easy, let's look at some basic survival tools.

Cooking Survival Tools

You really don't need designer cookware to make healthy, satisfying meals. If you're budget savvy, as I am, Walmart or the local dollar store will suffice for your basic kitchen necessities. If you don't have these essentials already, invest in:

- A large nonstick skillet (for stir-frying, browning, and sautéing).
- A slow cooker. This is a noncook's best friend! Mix, cover, and come back for a warm, hearty meal.
- A big casserole dish. Can you say "leftovers"?
- A few medium to large cooking or mixing spoons.
- An easy mixer, such as a Magic Bullet. I love mine: easy to use, easy to clean.
- A can opener.
- A good, sharp cutting knife.
- Plenty of dried and/or fresh seasonings (see Bam! Kick Up the Flavor on page 59 and the complete list on pages 60 to 61).
- Plastic storage containers. You can save time by cooking double servings, and you'll need something to put them in!
- A nonstick muffin pan. No, you're not gonna eat muffins. It's for a breakfast frittata.
- A cutting board.
- A set of measuring spoons.
- Sets of liquid and dry measuring cups.

Thin Waist, Thick Wallet

Let's face it: It's much cheaper to fill your body with junk than it is to eat healthy, all-natural foods. You would think that a product with less chemicals and preservatives would cost less, but that's not the case. You can buy a sleeve of cookies for as little as a dollar, while a pound of apples will set you back almost $4. It sort of leaves you scratching your head, doesn't it?

So how do you buy wholesome foods without breaking the bank? I'm glad you asked!

If you're already a savvy shopper, good for you! I had to learn to shop on a budget the hard way.

The first thing I learned is not to shop in posh specialty health food stores. Are they pretty? Yes. Do they make you feel special, as if you're getting healthier by just shopping there? Sure do. Do they break your bank? You betcha! You don't need a pricey store to eat healthfully. Stick to chain grocery or convenience stores like Walmart, where you can get fresh meat, dairy, and produce for reasonable prices. If you're lucky enough to have a local farmers' market or co-op near you, check them out! You'll get very fresh produce at a fraction of the price.

Other tips to help you make healthy choices while stretching your food dollars include the following:[1]

- Watch the sales so that you can buy healthy foods at reduced prices.
- Clip coupons (check out www.southernsavers.com for printable coupons at most major retail chains).
- Watch and compare the unit prices. Buy the least expensive amount that you will use.
- Buy in bulk, *if* you will use it and can store it.
- Switch from brand names to generic store brands.
- Shop the periphery of the store, where the food is more healthful and fresher.
- Buy in season. Seasonal produce has more nutrients, tastes better, and even costs less.

You've Got to Work!

It's important to eat healthy foods, but the food going in is only part of the equation. You need to Blast, Firm, and Burn to build muscle and torch calories and fat.

As with anything else in life, you can approach your workouts with fire and vigor or you can waltz right through them as if you're on a Sunday stroll. If busting your butt is going to get you from point A (mom jeans) to point B (skinny jeans) quicker, why in the world would you ever decide to waltz through? I'm going to teach you how to set that cute little body of yours on *fire!*

Right now I want you to create a character for me in your head so that when I speak, you know it's me. Now, I would prefer a sultry voice to a squeaky, high-pitched one, but it's your head, so I'll leave it up to you. Every time you work out, I want you to hear that voice. I'm going to be asking, "Where you at?" No, not your 10-20 (CB radio speak for *location*)—I'm checking in on your intensity!

To measure intensity, I love to use what's called a Borg Rating of Perceived Exertion (RPE) Scale, which ranges from 0 (nothing) to 10 (beyond hard). The RPE is a mind-body connection, a scan of your senses. Perceived exertion is based on the rate of intensity at which you are exercising and how your body responds to it.

The feelings I want you to be aware of are increased heart rate, muscle fatigue, rate of breathing, amount of perspiration, and/or any dizziness or nausea you may be experiencing. Yes, it's subjective, but it's a fairly reliable estimate of how hard your body is working

Two people doing the same exact workout can have two totally different RPEs because of varying levels of fitness, so if you see someone running like a cheetah without breaking a sweat, don't worry. Your RPE is about *you.*

How to Use Your RPE Scale

As you're working out, that (hopefully) sultry, stern voice of mine is going to say, "Where you at, girl? Are you working hard or hardly working?" Then you're going to reply either vocally or in your head, "I'm at a 6!" (See the "RPE Scale" on the next page.)

When you answer me, I don't ever want to hear anything below a 5! If you're below a 5, you might as well go lie down, 'cause you're not in this to win it. On a scale from 1 to 10, 1 is sitting on the couch eating bonbons, and 10 is going so hard that you start to feel dizzy and/or nauseated. You should never be either. You want to fly around a 5 to an 8.

RPE SCALE

0 = Nothing: You're on the couch with a face full of chips.

1 = Almost nothing: You're painting your nails.

2 = Very, very light: You're walking to the mailbox.

3 = Fairly light: You're vacuuming for exercise.

4 = Light: You are on cruise control, riding a bike through the park and looking at the trees.

5 = Moderate: Now you're doing something that feels like exercise!

6 = Fairly hard: Wow, here comes the burn.

7 = Hard: It's getting uncomfortable in a good way.

8 = Very hard: Almost to your limit, but you're able to hang.

9 = Extremely hard: Starting to see stars. You don't know how much longer you can continue.

10 = Beyond hard: OMG, gonna puke! The room is spinning!

HOW TO TURN UP THE HEAT (See the "Too Easy?" suggestions after each exercise in Chapter 5)

Speed it up.

Take less rest or no rest between sets.

Add weight or resistance to the exercise.

Do the harder version of the exercise.

HOW TO DIAL IT BACK (See the "Too Hard?" suggestions after each exercise in Chapter 5)

Move slower.

Take longer rests between sets.

Do the easier version of the exercise.

Let's get rolling! Turn to Chapter 5 and start cranking out the Blast, Firm, and Burn workouts, baby!

Supercharge My Skinny

Go Back to Class

I love to take group fitness classes as much as I love to teach them! It's like girls' night out with weights, and you don't have to worry about your outfit or makeup. Endorphins take the place of booze, and the music is thumping as you move and groove. You're feeding off of one another's energy. It's my version of utopia.

Now, I must admit, not all group fitness classes are created equal. A class is only as good as the instructor and her music. But once you find a class style you like or the type of instructor that gets your motor cranking, you're cooking with gas, baby!

Don't know what kinds of classes are out there? That's why you have me. Head to your local health club or group fitness, yoga, or dance studio and check out one of the classes starting below to follow the Supercharge My Skinny plan.

Smooth

If thumping music and hot, sweaty bodies gyrating all over the place aren't your thing, you might want to try a yoga, bar, Pilates, or fusion class. These classes are normally nonaerobic and focus on toning your muscles through fluid movement. Even though you're not getting your heart rate up, you'll still burn a ton of calories—and stretch and flex your way into your skinny jeans.

Yoga: Yoga is like the Baskin-Robbins of group fitness classes: There are 31 flavors. Actually, I don't know what the exact count is, but there are a lot! Some are very spiritual, while others are very athletic. Some focus strictly on holding postures, while others focus on flow. Some emphasize body alignment and breathing. You need to taste-test and find out which flavor *you* like best.

Bar: Using the Bar Method is becoming the new rage in group fitness. You perform ballet-based toning exercises while actually using a ballet bar for most of the class. And I bet you thought it was called Bar because it was held in a nightclub. No such luck! Have you ever seen a ballerina with a flabby butt? I think not. See, going to the bar can be a good thing!

Pilates: Pilates also has many varieties. Some classes involve large pieces of equipment, like the Reformer, while in others, your body is the only equipment you need. Pilates is great for toning and strengthening your legs, thighs, and core. It sounds kind of soft, but you will definitely feel the burn! You'll learn moves like the Corkscrew (sorry for the wine reference). They look easy—but looks are deceiving. Your tummy will be on fire!

Fusion: These classes can be a mix of different styles of yoga and Pilates combined into one. Check out your local health club or group fitness studio to see which style(s) they offer.

Upbeat

Get ready to shake your moneymaker or kick a little butt! These classes have high energy and thumping music. It's a party!

Zumba: This exotic-sounding workout is Latin-based. You don't need to know how to dance, but you'd better leave your inhibitions at the door. You're gonna be shaking, grinding, and shimmying everything your momma gave you to hot Latin music. And you know what? Even if you're a complete prude, you're going to love it!

You'll learn dance moves like "salsa," the "sugarcane," and in some classes even a little hip-hop. Funny how moves that burn a huge number of calories are named after yummy-sounding foods. Hopefully they'll make you crave getting your groove on!

Indoor cycling (or spinning): In a typical Spin class, you'll spend 45 minutes to 1 hour on a stationary bike, usually in a dimly lit room with thumping music. Sounds kind of kinky, huh? This class is one of my favorites! It might be because I get to go into my own head—enter my own zone—but I also love how it makes my butt look. And I love the loud music. Whatever it is, I always keep coming back for more. Throughout the class, the instructor will give you direction on the amount of tension to add and how fast you should pedal, but ultimately it's up to you how hard you work. Spinning is a great workout for all fitness levels.

Tae Bo (or kickboxing): Where else can you burn a massive number of calories while feeling as if you're kicking someone's butt? What a great class, and what great therapy! Tae Bo uses all of the kicks and punches from martial arts and boxing to fun, upbeat music. It's a rush! You've got to try it!

OMG

Don't let these classes intimidate you; they only sound scary. All you need are the cojones to try them once, and you'll be back for more.

Boot camp: Boot camp sessions are huge right now. Most include running, calisthenics (like jumping jacks and burpees), and resistance training all in one workout. It's kind of like a school gym class packed with fun activities, but you'll be sweating up a storm.

TRX: TRX is actually the name of a suspension-training device that uses your own body weight for resistance. This is a great workout for muscle toning and strength building. Most health clubs are now offering TRX classes, so check one out for a fun and challenging workout.

Indoor rowing: This may sound intimidating, but it's actually very easy to get the hang of and is one of the best total-body workouts on the face of the Earth. You'll be working your legs, abs, and upper body, and it's all nonimpact. You can burn up to 1,000 calories in a 45-minute class! Just like with Spinning, you are in control of your own Erg (rowing machine). The teacher will give you instructions on how hard to pull with your arms and push with your legs, but the amount of effort you put in is ultimately up to you. Classes are normally taught with fun, upbeat music and are designed to make time feel as if it's flying by. So by all means, go row your boat! To find a class near you, check out www.concept2.com.

With all of that variety, you're bound to find a class that fits the Supercharge My Skinny plan, right? Now, what will you need to get going?

Before You Go

The gym or instructor will usually provide all necessary equipment. Just make sure you're in good athletic shoes and comfortable clothing (see Shopaholics, Unite! on page 44). All skill levels are welcome in most classes, but check the schedule to be sure. It will usually mention if the class isn't recommended for beginners.

The cost of classes will vary from facility to facility. You may need a gym membership, but most group fitness classes are included in the price of your membership. If your facility charges extra for classes, you might be able to purchase a punch card. Don't want to join a gym? Call around; a good number of health clubs today offer punch cards to be used exclusively for classes. You can also grab a Groupon (www.groupon.com), if they're available in your area, for a greatly discounted rate.

And remember your water!

The Can-Do Society

Change isn't always easy, and it's even harder when you're going it alone. At some point, all of us need a sidekick (or two or five). If you're like me and affirmation is your love language, you might need a whole army of people to keep you motivated and stroke your ego. Don't judge yourself; there is definitely power in numbers.

MOTIVATION NATION

The number one rule of building a Can-Do Society: You've got to motivate the troops. Kill them with excitement and enthusiasm! Make them want—no, desire; no, *crave!*—what you've got!

It is essential to have people believe in you, to encourage you, to rejoice in your successes and sniffle with you during your failures. There are also days when you need a workout buddy to help drag your butt out of the house to the gym.

I like to call these inspirational pals the Can-Do Society. Your society can be made up of anyone you choose: family members, co-workers, friends, friends of friends, or complete strangers on Facebook or Twitter. We are a social network–obsessed society. Why not use it to your advantage?

Building Your Society

Friends: Take some advice from the *queen* of suckering people into doing things that they wouldn't dream of doing—from taking up exercise for the first time to running half marathons and triathlons: Give your friends a copy of this book, and let them know how great it's going for you. Talk to them enthusiastically about what you're doing, and convince them that joining you would be a blast! An ounce of enthusiasm goes a long way. Bait them with excitement.

Family: Hurray for family: an instant support group! If you don't have family nearby, adopt your friends' family members. They won't mind sharing.

Friends of friends and family: It's like multilevel marketing. Ask two people to join you in your skinny jeans quest, and then have those two people ask two people to join you, and there you go. You've got your very own society!

Religious or social club: Ask and you shall receive. Have the leaders send out a workout-buddy request in the newsletter. Better yet, just ask people yourself!

Facebook: Facebook is my number one pick for building a Can-Do Society!

When I started building my Can-Do Society to support or join me in doing triathlons for charity, I started a Team TRI Pink Facebook page. At first it was only my close friends. Then, to my surprise, it didn't just grow; it *blew up!* All of my friends and their friends got on the page, and before I knew it, people from all over the world had jumped on. When I started the page in May 2009, I had about 80 friends. Within one year, my triathlon team and I had more than 600 friends from 15 countries!

That's the power of a social network to build a society. Don't want to start your own Can-Do Society page? Jump on board with ours! Go to www.facebook .com/sixweekstoskinnyjeans and click "Like." There's no easier way to join a Can-Do Society. And we love new friends!

Kids: Do you have kids? Do your kids have friends? Do those friends have moms? You have a society. Ask them to go for walks with you during your kids' practices, or meet them for other "mom time" athletic activities.

Craigslist: Post a workout-buddy ad on your area's Craigslist. As always, proceed with caution when requesting to meet with someone you don't know, but this can be a great way to reach out to potential Can-Do Society members.

Meet-up group: Go to www.meetup.com and start your very own fitness meet-up group, or, if you see one, join an existing group.

Tweet: If you're on Twitter, send out a workout-buddy SOS. Keep your followers pumped and updated about what you're doing. The more positive you are about your progress and your program, the more they'll want to be a part of it.

Blog: This is like tweeting, only a little more labor intensive. Tweets are little one-liners; blogging is like journaling. There are many free blogging Web sites out there, but my favorite is WordPress (www.wordpress.com). Once you've got your blog set up, invite your friends to get your blog feed. Through this vehicle, you can keep them thoroughly updated on your day-to-day progress. Be sure to include commonly searched phrases such as *weight loss, diet,* and *exercise* so that others can find you through search engines. You can also start your own blog on www.amycotta.com.

Chat rooms and message boards: Type "weight loss chat room" or "diet message board" into any search engine and your screen will be filled with other virtual friends in your shoes. Decide which group best suits your taste and join the conversation.

My Web site, www.amycotta.com: And don't forget to make friends there, too! We would love to meet you and encourage you.

Okay, so you've got your society. Now your job is to ask them for support. *And* offer them support in return. Convince them to join you. Remember that the more excited you are, the more society members you will gain. Go get 'em, tiger!

Go Right Now and Start Facebooking and Tweeting Your Journey!

SKINNY 411
The average person consumes 9 pounds of food additives per year. Yuck!

THE **SKINNY**—*From Someone Who's Been There*

"I must say, it takes a ton of veggies to equal any real calories if you aren't putting crap on the veggies when you fix them."
—*Liza, Skinny Jeans Rock Star (page 115)*

Warning: Not everyone is going to love the new-and-improved, go-getter you. Read more about this issue in Mean Girls, page 182.

Think Yourself Thin

I knew that title would get your attention! Wouldn't it be great if all you had to do was snap your fingers and—*poof!*—you were a size 2? We all know that weight loss isn't nearly that easy, but there is some truth to thinking yourself thin. Your attitude and perspective are absolutely essential to dominating the Skinny Jeans program. Your thoughts are what will guide you to success or to failure. If you're in the wrong state of mind, you won't stick it out through the exercises or follow the eating plan.

Garbage in your mind = Garbage in your mouth

Sometimes your biggest saboteur can be the enemy within. That's right: I'm talking about *you!* Power thinkers from Jack Canfield to Deepak Chopra say that the average person has about 60,000 thoughts per day (too bad negative thinking doesn't burn calories; we'd all be a size 2!) and that 80 percent of those thoughts are negative. Anthony Robbins's book *Awaken the Giant Within* (yes, I'm a self-help nerd) tells us that there are more than 3,000 words in American English that relate to human emotions, and of those words, 2,086 of them are negative!

So what does all of this tell us? That the average person thinks 80 percent negatively? That two times out of three, the average American chooses a negative word out of the hat? Yes, maybe. But you are not average! Average people have little willpower. Average people don't stick to the plan. And average people can't button up their skinny jeans.

While we may feel that we live in a negative world, it's up to us to go against the grain. Taking personal responsibility for what you do, think, feel, say, and eat is all a part of inducing change.

What would you do if your computer got a virus? I'm assuming you'd clean the virus off your system so that your computer ran properly. Think about negative feelings and self-deprecation as a computer virus of the brain. You've got to clean out your hard drive and replace it with clean programming. No one can do it but you.

Skinny Fiction: Muscle Turns into Fat When You Stop Working Out

This one always gives me a huge chuckle. Let me assure you that it is humanly impossible. Fat and muscle are two completely different types of tissue, and one cannot genetically morph into the other. If that were true, you could turn fat into muscle and everyone who ever lifted a weight would look like a young Arnold Schwarzenegger—jacked and without a single ounce of fat.

Most fitness-illiterate people believe this myth because either they or someone they know stopped working out and got fatter. Here's what really happened. You "used to" exercise regularly and eat a healthy, low-calorie diet. Your body had a beautiful, toned shape with very little noticeable fat. Then one day you stopped exercising. Your lean, metabolism-boosting muscle started diminishing, and as your diet got worse, all the excess calories you consumed got stored as fat. As you gained weight, your fat cells increased in size while your muscle cells decreased in size (or atrophied). As you'll learn in Chapter 9, a pound of muscle takes up less space than a pound of fat. You ended up with curves in all the wrong places and were suddenly wearing jeans three sizes larger.

See? One didn't magically turn into the other. When you stopped working out, calorie-hungry muscle waved bye-bye, and fat cells came to stay. I don't have to tell you that the curves you get from muscle are much prettier than curves from fat, so go work out and burn those calories, girl!

TALK YOURSELF UP

Scientific research has shown that positive self-talk works if you put it into practice, and when these words are accompanied by an emotion or an image (like seeing yourself thin or enjoying exercise), positive thoughts will stay stored in your brain even longer.

In the upcoming weeks, you're going to have a little homework to do to keep your attitude in check. Remember you've got to get that **A** so that you can keep the **D** and **E** that lead to the skinny. So don't blow off these assignments!

Turn the Beat Around

Let's jump right in. From this point forward, every time you feel or want to say something negative, I want you to stop dead in your tracks. Immediately—and this is key—change and put a positive spin on what you are thinking, are about to say, or have just said.

Below are some examples of negative self-talk.

VIRUS	ANTIVIRUS
I can't.	I can and I will.
I'm too tired.	I have the energy.
I don't have time.	I make time.
Exercise is too hard.	I love being active and healthy.
Losing weight is impossible.	I lose weight easily.
I hate dieting.	I like making healthy, satisfying food choices.

Homework!

What negativity do you have that needs to be taken out with the trash? I want you to use the space below to write it all out. Be honest. If you're just making stuff up to get to the next page faster, you will miss the whole lesson. Okay, move!

Bad _____

_____

_____

_____

_____

Replace With _____

_____

_____

_____

_____

My Skinny Check-In

☐ I cleaned out the pantry and refrigerator.

☐ I shopped for Skinny Jeans foods.

☐ I started logging my eating and exercise.

☐ I looked for members of my Can-Do Society.

☐ I followed workouts as planned.

☐ I Supercharged My Skinny activities!

☐ I kept a positive attitude!

Skinny Jeans
ROCK ST★R

Before: Size 9   After: Size 4

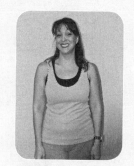

Name: Itzel

Age: 46

Occupation: Court reporter and chef

Children: 2

Pounds lost: 19.6

What I was afraid of: Nothing. I was determined to do everything and stick to the program 100 percent.

What I liked: I didn't feel hungry. Actually, at the beginning it was rather hard to eat all 1,500 calories!

What I learned: Vanity is a powerful motivation when it comes to losing weight. Never say never, and I mean never! If you want big rewards, you need to make big sacrifices. When you eat healthy, you can lose weight without getting hungry. The stupid scale is a big, fat, lousy liar; your clothes are not! Your friends might love you, but they can also be enablers, and that is not a good thing when you are on a diet. Stay away from them if you must.

What I want to share: This is the best weight loss program!

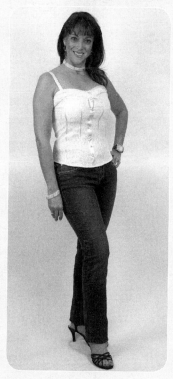

Chapter 3

Week 2: WELCOME TO HELL WEEK

My Skinny Action Plan

☐ Replenish my Skinny Jeans foods (if needed).

☐ Drink eight to ten 8-ounce glasses of water every day!

☐ Log my eating and exercise.

☐ Recruit workout buddies.

☐ Don't miss workouts!

☐ Do my attitude homework.

Welcome to Hell Week

Okay, so how are you feeling? Are you hanging in there? This is the toughest week of the 6-week program. The honeymoon is over, the lack of carbs is probably making you irritable, and you're likely feeling the effects of sugar withdrawal. It's okay. That's normal, and it does get better. Just remember that the things you are missing and craving are the things that got you where you are.

Once you get through this week, the next 4 will seem like smooth sailing. Your cravings are going to disappear, and you're going to be feeling and looking awesome! Keep pushing, keep working hard, and keep a good attitude. You have a choice: This week can be complete and utter hell, or you can make it a great week, a mountain to climb and conquer. I suggest that you keep climbing, girl; carbs and sanity are on the way!

Skinny Jeans Calendar: Week 2

D = Diet; E = Exercise; A = Attitude (food log)   SMS = Supercharge My Skinny

MON	TUE	WED	THUR	FRI	SAT	SUN
☐ **D** Ignite ☐ **E** Off ☐ **A** Journal ☐ SMS	☐ **D** Ignite ☐ **E** Blast ☐ **A** Journal ☐ SMS	☐ **D** Ignite ☐ **E** Firm ☐ **A** Journal ☐ SMS	☐ **D** Ignite ☐ **E** Burn ☐ **A** Journal ☐ SMS	☐ **D** Ignite ☐ **E** Off ☐ **A** Journal ☐ SMS	☐ **D** Ignite ☐ **E** Blast ☐ **A** Journal ☐ SMS	☐ **D** Ignite ☐ **E** Firm ☐ **A** Journal ☐ SMS

Are You Really Hungry?

I love scales. No, not the kind you stand on: Those can be evil when used too often! I'm talking about *perception scales*, which make you stop, think, and scan your body for feedback. The Skinny Jeans Rate of Perceived Hunger (RPH) Scale below will help you decide if you're really hungry or if you need to be pulled away from the table.

SKINNY JEANS RPH SCALE

1 = **Famished:** You are beyond hungry—ready to eat your arm off!

2 = **Extremely hungry:** You're eyeing little kids' lunches.

3 = **Hungry:** Your tummy is growling, playing show tunes.

4 = **First sign of hunger:** There is a little rumble in your jungle.

5 = **Content:** You're good to go, neither full nor hungry.

6 = **Feel somewhat full:** Your tank is three-quarters full.

7 = **Full:** You could walk away right now; no longer feeling hungry.

8 = **Very full:** There isn't any more room in your tummy.

9 = **Stuffed!** You're thinking about unbuttoning your pants!

10 = **Beyond stuffed!** You're feeling sick, wondering why someone didn't stop you.

On the RPH Scale, the goal is to make sure that you are never at 1 or 10. You want to hang out somewhere between 4 and 7, which means you'll need to eat small, frequent meals throughout the day. This allows your body to use the food you're taking in as energy without having leftover calories stored away as fat. Going too long without eating is just as bad as overeating. It messes with your metabolism, and you'll be so famished that you'll be tempted to stop at a drive-thru, pick up a candy bar, or worse.

The key here is *not* to go hungry for so long that you'll be tempted to eat outside of your Skinny Jeans eating plan. That's why you must learn to constantly read your level of hunger and make sure you are prepared with healthy snacks when hunger does strike. Pack a snack bag the day before with more than enough of what you're *supposed* to be eating.

That'll help you get through the day, but sometimes you need help just getting through a meal, right? Pop quiz: You're eating a meal, and it's the greatest-tasting food you've ever had. The portion size is large, and you're feeling full. What do you do? No, you don't keep eating until it's all gone. You walk away from the table! Yes, you heard me: Stop eating. When you feel satisfied, just stop eating! I don't care how good it tastes. If it's that scrumptious, it will taste just as good as a leftover. Get up, grab a container, and save that food for later!

Stuffed tummy = Stuffed pants!

You do want those skinny jeans to fit, don't you? Walk away!

Drink, Baby, Drink

Do you enter a blank fog in the middle of the day? Does every step you take feel like a chore? Does it take everything you've got to keep off the couch? You may think you need to eat for energy, but in reality, you're probably thirsty. Yep, sister, you need to refill your tank. Even mild dehydration can cause afternoon fatigue, and because dehydration lowers your metabolism, eating is definitely not the right choice. Downing some good old H_2O will turn you back around. (If you're dragging all day long, see the section The F-Word, page 46.)

If you're like me, you love your coffee in the morning and your tea or diet cola in the afternoon. Unfortunately, these caffeinated drinks are also diuretics that help flush water out of your body, making your need to hydrate properly even greater. Try to keep it down to one or two diet sodas or cups of coffee per day (see Give Me Coffee or Give Me Death! on page 162).

And you're going to want to be chugging that water when you hear this next statistic! Researchers are not really sure why, but they've found that drinking at least eight glasses of water a day can burn off almost 35,000 calories a year! That's 10 pounds of weight loss! And they've even found that cold water works best because warming the water to body temperature burns calories, too.[1]

The moral of the story: Drink water, whether you're thirsty or not. In fact, don't even let yourself get thirsty, because that means you're past the point of mild dehydration. I know you want to burn those extra calories and avoid those afternoon slumps, so keep a full glass or bottle of water at your desk, in your bag, or in your car at all times!

Label Me Confused

Although I don't particularly enjoy grocery shopping, I'm a huge supermarket label reader. I believe you need to compare food labels of anything that is pre-packaged because, let's face it, not all man-made food is created equal.

Food manufacturers have caught on that people are reading labels more these days. A few years ago, you wouldn't have seen health claims on the front of your favorite breakfast cereals, but today you'll see boxes claiming that their contents will help you lose weight!

This product box is an advertisement piece with what we in the infomercial business call the wow factor. The wow factor is that one thing that makes your product so unique that a consumer just *has* to have it. Special K's wow factor is its claim that you will lose weight if you eat this cereal. Really? That's all I have to do? And all these years I've been exercising to keep the weight off . . .

Just because a product claims to be healthy doesn't make it so. Don't ever trust the front of the package! Skip over the colorful pictures and word art and look at that plain black-and-white rectangle on the back: the Nutrition Facts. This little chart has all the facts you need to know.

The first thing to be aware of on a food label is the serving size. All the other specifications—like calories, fat, and sodium—are based on the serving size, not the entire package, and some products will make the serving size tiny in order to keep the fat and calories low. So think about how much you will actually be eating in one sitting before you decide that the product is healthy enough to buy!

The calories listed are also for the serving size only—not the entire package. Of course, some items may say "Serving size: 1 bar." But the bottom line is that serving size is very important in determining the number of calories in a meal.

While the total number of calories is listed, the amount of carbohydrate, fats, and protein will help you determine what constitutes the total number of calories. Carbohydrate, fats, and protein are listed by weight in grams.

1 gram of carbohydrates = 4 calories
1 gram of protein = 4 calories
1 gram of fat = 9 calories

So if a serving size contains 5 grams of protein, 20 of the total calories would come from protein.

The fat content in foods is usually broken down into total fat and saturated fat (and trans fat, if there is any). Saturated fat, most often derived from animal products, is what you need to stay away from. Eating too much saturated fat can lead to clogged arteries and a rise in your LDL (bad) cholesterol. This is why I suggest staying away from fatty meat sources, full-fat dairy products, and of course processed snack foods like cookies and doughnuts. Good sources of healthy, unsaturated fats are olive oil, olives, nuts, nut butters, avocados, and fatty fish such as salmon and trout. Your body requires fat to function, and it will keep you feeling full, so don't cut it out completely. The American Heart Association suggests keeping your total fat intake to about 25 to 35 percent of your daily calories. To determine the number of fat calories in a food, use a method like this:

1 serving of Jif peanut butter = 2 tablespoons

Calories = 190

Fat = 16 grams

1 gram of fat = 9 calories

16 grams x 9 calories = 144 calories in fat

The list of ingredients on food labels can be equally important in determining the nutritional benefit of a product because they are listed in order of their weight per serving. For example, if high-fructose corn syrup is listed first, the product is going to be a high-sugar, high-carbohydrate food, so stay away! Remember, high-GI foods break down quickly and release glucose rapidly into your system—causing weight gain and curtailing your Skinny Jeans efforts.

When you read a food label, note that there are many manufacturer terms that translate directly into fat and sugar.

FATS

Hydrogenated vegetable shortening

Lard

Lecithin

Oil

Palm kernel oil

Triglycerides

SUGARS

Corn syrup

Dextrose

Fructose

Lactose

Maltose

Sucrose

Truth in Labels

Fortunately, the use of terms such as "low fat" and "low calorie" is now heavily regulated for consistency in meaning so that manufacturers can no longer sell under false pretenses. But that doesn't mean you can drop your guard. When you think you're cutting out one bad ingredient, you're usually just adding more of something else that you don't want. For example, fat-free products are usually filled with sugar or sodium to make up for the taste that's lost when the fat is removed. Fruit juice cocktails are another misleading product. They're in the juice aisle, they look like juice, and they smell like juice, but they usually contain only about 10 percent real juice. Make sure you check out the list of other ingredients: Usually these beverages aren't much healthier than Kool-Aid.

Below is a list of some supermarket lingo with true definitions. Familiarize yourself with these terms, and you'll be better armed to make healthier choices.[2]

Calorie free: Fewer than 5 calories per serving.

Sugar free: Less than 0.5 grams of sugar per serving.

Fat free: Less than 0.5 grams of total fat per serving.

Low fat: 3 grams or fewer total fat grams per serving.

Low saturated fat: 1 gram or less per serving.

Low sodium: Fewer than 140 milligrams per serving.

Very low sodium: Fewer than 35 milligrams per serving.

THE **SKINNY**—*From Someone Who's Been There*

"Logging the food became habit and was a huge eye opener. Shocking, in fact!"

—*Anne, Skinny Jeans Rock Star (page 156)*

Low cholesterol: Fewer than 20 milligrams per serving.

Low calorie: 40 calories or fewer per serving.

Lean: Fewer than 10 grams of fat, 4 grams of saturated fat, and 95 milligrams of cholesterol per serving and per 100 grams of meat, poultry, or seafood.

Extra lean: Fewer than 5 grams of fat, 2 grams of saturated fat, and 95 milligrams of cholesterol per serving and per 100 grams of meat, poultry, or seafood.

High: One serving contains 20 percent or more of the Daily Value for that nutrient.

Good source: One serving contains 10 to 19 percent of the Daily Value for that nutrient.

Reduced: A nutritionally altered product that contains 25 percent less of a nutrient or calories than the regular product.

Less: A food (that may or may not be altered) that contains 25 percent less of a nutrient or calories than the regular product or food.

Light: A nutritionally altered product that contains one-third fewer calories or half of the fat of the regular food or product. It can also mean that the sodium content of a low-calorie, low-fat food has been reduced by half.

More: One serving contains at least 10 percent more of the Daily Value of a nutrient than the regular food or product.

A few other common terms that might need some explanation are:

From concentrate: Juices from concentrate should have the same nutritional value as the original juice product. *Concentrate* means that at some point, much of the water was removed for easier shipping, and water was added back in to reconstitute the original consistency of the juice. (Think frozen orange juice.)

Sugar alcohol (or polyols): These naturally occurring sweeteners are often used as sugar substitutes because they provide anywhere from half to one-third the calories of regular sugar. Also, unlike regular sugar, they don't cause an immediate jump in blood sugar. Some common sugar alcohols are mannitol, sorbitol, xylitol, lactitol, isomalt, maltitol, and hydrogenated starch hydrolysates (HSH).[3] Consuming sugar alcohols in high volumes can cause abnormal gas, discomfort, and diarrhea.

Multigrain, whole grain: These terms are *not* interchangeable. *Whole grain* means that all parts of the grain kernel—the bran, germ, and endosperm—are used in the making of the product. *Multigrain*, however, means that a food contains *more than one type* of grain. Whole grain foods—listed as "whole grain," "whole wheat," and "whole oats"—are the healthier choice.[4]

Warning: Most fat-free products contain high amounts of sugar in order to make up for the loss of taste from the fat. On the flip side, low-sugar products usually have a higher fat content. So read labels and choose wisely!

Eco-Terms Defined

Our world is growing more green and eco-conscious by the day. Trendy food stores selling the latest environmentally friendly and organic products are popping up everywhere. These politically correct green stores seem to have their own lingo, and if you are eco-illiterate like I am, you might feel a bit baffled and overwhelmed when trying to shop at them. Starting below, you'll find some of the most commonly used eco-terms.[5]

American grassfed: After animals are weaned, they eat only grass and forage (never grain). Growth hormones are prohibited, and if an animal has to take antibiotics, it is removed from the program. (A third party verifies this claim.)

USDA organic: Certified by the National Organic Program, these products are at least 95 percent organic, meaning no pesticides, fertilizers, hormones, antibiotics, radiation, or genetic engineering.

Fair-trade certified: Again, pesticides and genetically modified organisms (GMOs) are not allowed, but this term goes beyond the product itself to the farmers who provide it. The farmers of these products are ensured safe working conditions and fair wages and prices for crops. Plus, their businesses invest back into their communities.

Free range: According to the USDA, this label applies only to chicken—and can mean as little as 5 minutes of "outdoor access" a day. Plus, free-range chickens may still share small, confined living space with caged chickens. On the flip side, caged chickens are kept in coops 24-7 without any free movement, and some people feel that the quality of the product is truly diminished.

Whether your food claims to make you skinny or save the Earth, don't necessarily become a victim of the hype. Know the facts, and choose your groceries based on the nutritional info, not the bold, flashy print on the front of the package. And both phases of this Skinny Jeans eating plan were purposely designed to steer you almost entirely toward foods with no labels at all! You don't need a big red sticker to tell you that an apple is a healthy choice.

Skinny Fiction: Exercise Will Make Me Look Bulky

No, a big butt and flabby gut will make you look bulky!

Cardio and strength training will help you look thinner and healthier while you burn an amazing number of calories. (See "Skinny Fiction: Muscle Weighs More Than Fat" on page 186).

Female bodies, unlike male ones, are not designed to bulk up. Yes, some women gain muscle faster and easier than others. But no matter how much weight you lift, you will never get bigger muscles than your boyfriend or husband. It is impossible with our genetic makeup. Women naturally have lower levels of testosterone (the muscle-building hormone) than men, so we can lift weights just as hard as they do but never get to be their size or strength. So don't worry. Keep working out, and if you want to challenge yourself by lifting heavier weights, go for it! You won't turn into a bodybuilder!

Shopaholics, Unite!

It's time to gear up and fill that closet with some workout clothes, baby! You should keep in mind that when it comes to fitness, it's about function, not fashion. You're gonna move and you're gonna sweat, so you need clothes and shoes that work with you, not against you—and that you don't mind getting worn and dirty!

Shoes

First, take care of your feet by investing in a good athletic sneaker. You will especially need them for Supercharge My Skinny activities such as running, walking, or taking a group fitness class (some of the Blast and Firm exercises can be performed barefoot).

Choosing the right shoe is essential. An incorrectly fitting sneaker can make any kind of exercise—even just walking around the house—miserable. Finding the proper style and fit for your foot's shape and size, the way you walk, and the type of exercise you'll be doing will make all the difference in your comfort, stamina, and persistence in workouts. Exercise itself is tough, and it will be a lot tougher with blisters on your feet. Let's look at some ways that will help you find that Cinderella fit.

- **Go shoe shopping late in the day.** Women's bodies have this annoying little habit of swelling, and our feet are no exception. As they swell throughout the day, a comfortable early-morning purchase can turn into a potentially painful one by dinnertime.

- **Stand when you're measured!** Unlike your butt, which expands when you sit down, your feet expand when you stand up. So always stand when getting your feet measured to ensure that your foot is fully extended.

- **Not all feet are created equal.** Try on both shoes when you're wearing running socks, and choose the size that fits your larger foot best.

- **Size matters.** Your big toe should be a thumbnail width from the top end of the shoe. The salesclerk should be able to help you out with this. If the shoes don't feel cushy and wonderful in the store, *don't buy them*. Try another brand.

Sports Bra

Next, you'll want to keep your girls under lock and key with a high-quality sports bra. Just take my advice, and try it before you buy it!

- If the bra straps pull on your shoulders or the bra feels like an elephant is sitting on your chest, it's too small. If you buy one that's too small, you'll end up paying the price later with neck and shoulder pain.

- If the bra feels good, perform a few jumping jacks in the dressing room. (Yes, I'm serious.) If you are bouncing around uncomfortably, your bra is too big. But if you feel fully supported, it's a winner!

- When in doubt, let the salesclerk help you out with proper sizing and style selection.

Material

Workout-clothing manufacturers have improved their products by leaps and bounds in the last few years, with some very effective moisture-wicking, low-friction materials. Unlike cotton, which holds in perspiration and odor, moisture-wicking materials pull the perspiration from your body, keeping you clean, cool, and dry.

So how do you know if your purchase is moisture wicking? It will most likely have a hanging tag boasting its ability to keep you dry during activity. Major players in the athletic-garment business, such as Under Armour, Reebok, Nike, and Puma, all offer wicking products ranging from shirts to pants to socks to hats. Most of these brands work with CoolMax, a blend of synthetic fabrics that comes in different performance levels for hot- and cold-weather training. If your purchase doesn't have a hanging tag specifying that it is moisture wicking, look at the inside tag. Most wicking materials are made up of some sort of polyester, nylon, or spandex blend.

Don't Forget Your Drawers

Make sure your workout shorts or pants fit and that you can move comfortably in them. If you plan to be jogging, make sure the legs are loose enough to prevent painful rubbing. Moisture wicking is also a major plus down there.

The F-Word

Even with the perfect diet and the best exercise gear, you're probably going to feel some fatigue during your Skinny Jeans journey. I know there's nothing worse than feeling like a sack of bones with zero energy, where every step is like a major chore, and all you want to do is fall into a bed face-first. However, you can work to prevent fatigue from cramping your style by knowing exactly what causes it.

Fatigue Busters

1. **Get plenty of sleep.** I know that's easier said than done (and I have the dark circles to prove it). Research suggests that the average person needs between 7 and 8 hours of sleep a night. I need a good 9 or 10 to be fully alert and productive, so don't fret if 7 just isn't cutting it!

2. **Eat enough calories.** Okay, I realize the irony here. You're on a "diet," and you're restricting calories, but eating under your daily allotment will zap your energy levels. Pay careful attention during the Ignite phase, when you're eating mostly low-calorie vegetables and lean protein. Those calories need to add up!

3. **Stay hydrated.** It bears repeating. Even a slight bout of dehydration can cause major fatigue.

4. **Be aware of food allergies.** If your fatigue gets worse after you eat a certain type of food, you could have a slight allergy to it. If this is the case, you should talk with your doctor or dietitian to set the best course of action.

5. **Keep up with your workouts.** Get tired now to prevent more fatigue later. Research shows that a lack of exercise can turn you into a sloppy mess on the couch. The more you move, the more energy you'll have.

If you've done all the above and you just can't seem to shake it, girl, you could be anemic—meaning you have low iron. Talk to your doctor. A simple blood test can check your iron levels, and something as simple as a multivitamin/mineral supplement with iron could solve the problem.

Supercharge My Skinny

Swim for Sanity!

I love swimming, but it hasn't always been that way. Not long ago, I couldn't even swim across the pool. I soon realized what I had been missing! Not only is swimming great exercise, but it also relieves stress and is gentle on your body. I'm totally addicted! If you're a swimmer, you know exactly what I mean.

Corrections to Your Objections

I can't swim. Take lessons to learn the basics. Once you are able to stay afloat on your own, you can use fins, a kickboard, or a pool buoy to help you become even more competent. Don't worry about looking like a kid with a floaty: These are all training aids that swimmers use regularly. The key here is just to move! Get yourself across the pool, rest, and then get back. YouTube is full of great videos showing different swim drills that you can do, using training aids if you can't swim. Also consider using a flotation belt and running in deep water or just running in shallow water. Swimming and running in water are great alternatives to running if you have knee or hip issues. It's also a harder workout because of the water resistance.

People at the pool are going to judge me. I dealt with this myself. I didn't want to be seen in my swimsuit, and I thought the lifeguards were thinking, "Great; I'm going to have to pull this lady out of the water!" But really, everyone else is too busy with their own lives to care what you look like or how well you swim. It's all in your head.

Swimming laps is boring. If you approach it with a negative attitude, you certainly won't have fun! For me, swimming has become a form of meditation. It's just me and the water, and I find myself craving that alone time.

Swimming Benefits

It does the body good. Swimming helps increase flexibility and muscular and cardiovascular endurance. Water is denser than air and adds about 12 times more resistance. Because it takes more work to move through water, you'll be getting an awesome workout!

It's low impact. Swimming doesn't put the same stress on your muscles and joints that other forms of exercise do. This means that you can work really hard in the water, but you'll get out feeling great!

It's cheaper than therapy. Because swimming is so free of distraction, it allows you to focus on your breathing, your stroke, or nothing at all. You can just let your mind go on autopilot. Take my word on this one: Swimming has kept me from going postal on more than one occasion. After a good swim, you will leave the pool feeling mentally refreshed and recharged.

What you need to know before you go: If you're going to get your head in the water and swim, I suggest getting a cap and goggles to help protect your gorgeous locks and peepers. You'll also need a towel and flip-flops to protect your feet from the wet and germy pool deck and locker-room floors. If you have just learned to swim, I would recommend you get swim fins to keep you buoyant and in control. Most pools will have kickboards, pool buoys, and flotation belts for your use. If you want to buy your own, you can usually pick up a pair of fins or a flotation belt for around $25. A kickboard or a pool buoy will set you back about $15. The cost to use a lap pool (if you don't belong to a gym or other swimming facility) will vary from center to center.

End the Excuses

It gets a little crowded inside my head sometimes. I definitely have multiple personalities when it comes to training my clients.

First, there's the supportive Cheerleader. She's the perky, encouraging friend who will love you and cheer you on, no matter what. She'll hold your hand and cry with you when the going gets tough. She'll wipe your tears and tell you, "Everything's gonna be okay." She'll believe in you, even when you don't believe in yourself. And then the butt-kicking, Evil Personal Trainer busts in. She'll growl at you to suck it up and quit your whining. She'll give you *something to cry about!* Like a drill sergeant crossed with a pit bull, she'll order you to quit being a crybaby, shut up, and get to work.

It's a battle of wills between those two.

The Cheerleader yells, "Good try!"

The Trainer barks, "There's no such thing as *trying*—you either do something or you don't!"

Unfortunately, we need them both. Fortunately for you, I *am* both.

A Word from the Cheerleader

Nobody's perfect. Life happens. At some point we're all going to struggle; we're all going to have a rotten day and make some not-so-healthy choices. It's called being human. It happens to us all. The difference between success and failure is how you handle those bumps in the road.

A Word from the Evil Trainer

Seriously, how hard is it to plan your meals, eat well, and work out for a measly 45 minutes a day? You will get 100 percent of what you put into your plan. If you half-ass it, that's how much success you'll have. You want results? Results require action, not excuses!

The Realist

Though I demonstrate those two extremes, I am also a realist. I know that life can happen, and rarely does anything go exactly as planned. Don't get me wrong here; I am not—I repeat, not—giving you permission to eat yourself off the reservation because you're working out, or to skip the workouts because you're eating well. But if you do happen to stumble, don't sit on the ground whining about it. Get back up! Start again!

We all fall sometimes, but there are no excuses for quitting.

Excuse Busters from the Evil Trainer

1. **I don't have time to exercise.** Really? Do you watch TV? Do you constantly log on to Facebook or Twitter? You have time!

2. **I ate something bad, so I might as well go ahead and eat whatever I want today.** No! Don't follow one mistake with another. Cut your losses while you can and get back on track ASAP!

3. **It's too expensive to eat healthy.** Where do you shop? As I mentioned in Chapter 2, you don't have to shop at high-end health food stores to get fresh, nutritious food. I buy all of my vegetables at one of those discount stores where you bag your own groceries. The selection is great, and the prices are reasonable.

4. **My spouse isn't being supportive.** Get a new spouse! (Just joking.) Once your spouse starts to see your physical and emotional improvements, he'll come around.

5. **My kids' schedule is taking too much of my time.** Do you drive your kids to sports and stay there while they practice or play? Don't sit on your fanny— do something, anything! Do your Skinny Jeans workouts, walk, jog, *move!*

6. **Working out isn't any fun!** Your perception will dictate your mood. If you see exercise as a chore, it will be a chore. Don't look at it as something you have to do; look at it as something you want to do. Go do something that puts a smile on your face. Go take a hike or dance class with a friend. Doing Supercharge My Skinny activities will help remind you that there is more to exercise than just squats and crunches.

7. **Work is taking up too much of my time.** See excuse number one!

8. **I feel guilty. I should be taking care of my family instead of myself.** How can you take care of your family if your self-esteem is low and you are out of shape and unhealthy? Being a fit, active wife and mother is the best gift you could ever give your spouse and children.

9. **It's that time of the month; I just can't bear to work out.** We all have the curse. You can't let it stop you. Unless you are medically unable to move, pop a Midol and get up!

S— or Get Off the Pot

How many times have you wished you could change your body, your diet, or your exercise habits? How many times have you started to change your diet and exercise habits, only to go back to your old ways? Indecisiveness and lack of dedication will kill your dreams! There is only one way to change anything: You've just got to do it! Or, as my mom would so eloquently put it, "S— or get off the pot."

In order to make lasting change, you've got to get uncomfortable. You've got to demand more of yourself and for yourself. Commit right now to settling for nothing less than your best! Raise your standards!

What is your goal for the end of this 6-week journey? What pants size do you want to be in? What do you want your scale to say? Do you want to feel better? Be healthier? Are you dying to rock a designer dress at your high school reunion? Be specific about what you want.

With that said, you also have to be realistic. I do believe you can achieve *any-thing* you set your mind to. But if you're in a size 16 today, you're not going to fit into a size 2 in 6 weeks. I'm a good trainer, and you're awesome, but neither one of us is a magician. Set a realistic goal. If you surpass it, that's even better!

Homework Time!

MY GOALS ARE

Jean size: _____ Weight: _____

Other: _____

_____

Now, what are you no longer going to accept or tolerate about your life? Your fitness? What do you aspire to be? This is part of your program, girl. Don't just sit there—write it down!

_____

_____

_____

_____

If you're not going to make a 100 percent commitment to yourself, you might as well go ahead and use this book as a coaster. Because that's all it's going to end up being: something that lies around your house, taking up space, collecting dust.

Remember the DEA (diet, exercise, attitude) from earlier? You've got to get that A down, or D and E will not last long. You've got to change your attitude and your limited beliefs, or this book isn't worth much more than the paper it's printed on.

Where's Your Head?

What was the state of your D (diet) before you started this journey? What are you going to do to make sure you don't backslide? What about E (exercise)? Did you have an exercise routine before starting this program? What are you going to do to turn it up a notch? How good is your current A (attitude)? What steps will you take to make sure your attitude is stronger than your old negative thoughts and habits? Ponder these thoughts and then use the space provided below to write down your answers.

_____

_____

_____

_____

_____

_____

_____

_____

My Skinny Check-In

☐ I replenished my food.

☐ I stayed hydrated.

☐ I kept track of my eating and exercise.

☐ I looked for workout buddies.

☐ I didn't miss any workouts!

☐ I did my attitude homework.

Skinny Jeans
ROCK ST☆R

Before: Size 14   After: Size 12

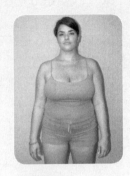

Name: Leah

Age: 25

Occupation: Marketing manager

Children: None

Pounds lost: 12

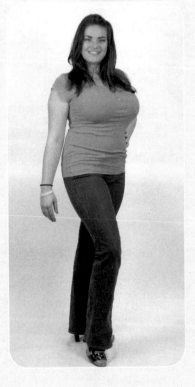

What I was afraid of: I was beyond ecstatic for the journey to begin. However, I had lingering negative thoughts in the back of my mind. I knew the program worked, but I wondered if my body would remember how to lose weight.

What I learned: This diet-and-exercise plan will work if you follow it! If you do not have success, it is not because the plan doesn't work. It is because you cheated or didn't follow the routine. You will reap what you sow.

What I want to share: Take advantage of group support (Facebook—the 6-week group especially). The Web site www.myfitnesspal.com is a great way to track calories and exercise. The exercises are for real … ain't no joke! They could be done in your living room, and they didn't take too long. Depending on how many breaks I took, I could get them done pretty quickly. The exercises were effective, and I loved the variety of having three different routines.

Chapter 4

Week 3: YOU'RE HALFWAY THERE, BABY!

My Skinny Action Plan

☐ Track my diet and exercise every day.

☐ Find more workout buddies!

☐ Supercharge My Skinny!

☐ Complete this week's attitude homework.

☐ Maintain a great attitude. I'm halfway there!

☐ Work the plan! Work the plan! Work the plan!

Hump Week!

Yes! You are halfway there, baby! At this point, there is nothing you can't accomplish.

I know you may still go to bed with visions of fruit and muffins dancing in your head. At least the muffins are now in your dreams and not on your hips. And next week, the fruit will be yours.

Now is *not* the time to falter. I know that when success is near, it's easy to say, "One little drink or one piece of chocolate isn't going to kill me. I've been good this long." Squelch those thoughts immediately; they can be the kiss of death.

Skinny Jeans Calendar: Week 3

D = Diet; E = Exercise; A = Attitude (food log)   SMS = Supercharge My Skinny

MON	TUE	WED	THUR	FRI	SAT	SUN
☐ **D** Ignite	☐ **D** Ignite	☐ **D** Ignite	☐ **D** Ignite	☐ **D** Ignite	☐ **D** Ignite	☐ **D** Ignite
☐ **E** Burn	☐ **E** Off	☐ **E** Blast	☐ **E** Firm	☐ **E** Burn	☐ **E** Off	☐ **E** Blast
☐ **A** Journal	☐ **A** Journal	☐ **A** Journal	☐ **A** Journal	☐ **A** Journal	☐ **A** Journal	☐ **A** Journal
☐ SMS	☐ SMS	☐ SMS	☐ SMS	☐ SMS	☐ SMS	☐ SMS

Don't give up. Don't give in. Stay strong, and stay the course. Part of this journey is about changing habits. Don't allow yourself to fall back into your old ways. You've made it too far to give up now!

Whatcha Eatin'?

Let's say—just hypothetically—that you've been on some crazy diet for, oh, say, more than 2 weeks now. (And you've been doing amazingly well, by the way.) It's been a rough week, but today is Friday. And a co-worker's birthday. And everyone just happens to be going to that irresistible Italian place for lunch. You've been killing yourself for 2 weeks now. You *so* deserve a break!

What does that nut Amy Cotta expect, anyway—for you to sit in the office all alone with your little brown bag? Besides, there's gotta be something healthy on the menu.

You can order something grilled, right?

Well, fast-forward 1 hour, one *grilled* Honey Balsamic Chicken, and 900 calories[1] later. You've blown your diet and you know it. Now you're mad at yourself.

Don't get me wrong. I love irresistible Italian restaurants as much as anyone, but restaurant eating is very dangerous to a girl striving for skinny jeans. Even the good choices can be deceptively bad. In order to make their food taste good, most restaurants cook with a lot of salt, oil, butter, cream—okay, I'll stop now. You get the point.

Enter the realist and cheerleader: I know the companionship of a girls' lunch is almost too tempting to pass up. But I'm only asking you for a 6-week commitment here, and you're doing so great! Please don't blow it now. If you do desperately want or feel you need to go, look over Restaurant Survival in Chapter 11, and be sure to keep your order selections within the Ignite phase: no bread, pasta, potatoes, or fruit.

Your best bet is to order a mixed salad with grilled chicken and ask for a light dressing or olive oil and vinegar on the side. You can also take along your own dressing (see "Salad Dressing Survival" below). I know it sounds odd, but do you want to look sane or skinny?

And you know the drill: Log every morsel that goes between those beautiful lips!

Enter the Evil Trainer: Don't go! The bottom line is that unless you're making it yourself, you just don't know what's going into your food. And right now, knowing what goes into your food—and, by extension, into your mouth—is of the upmost importance. Those skinny jeans depend on it.

SALAD DRESSING SURVIVAL (2-TABLESPOON SERVING SIZE)

Newman's Own Lighten Up Balsamic Vinaigrette: 45 calories

Kraft Roasted Red Pepper Vinaigrette: 35 calories

Wish-Bone Fat-Free Chunky Blue Cheese: 30 calories

Wish-Bone Fat-Free Ranch: 30 calories

Learn to Love the Lunch Box Again

Go back with me now a few years to elementary school. The smell of sharpened pencils and freshly waxed floors welcomed you back at the beginning of every new school year. And if you were like me, you walked across those shiny floors flashing your brand-new favorite-character lunch box—with a matching thermos to boot. Every weekday at lunch, I'd open that treasure chest and pull out the surprises that my mom or dad had lovingly packed for the day. Sometimes there'd even be a sweet note from them to make me smile.

We can rekindle that little lunch-box romance, can't we? If you haven't already, take some time and shop for a lunch box that you're going to love—really. You've got a favorite color, right? There's a lunch box in that color. Lucky for us, customized bags are pretty trendy right now. Just drop into one of your favorite boutiques or embroidery shops, or even Google "personalized lunch boxes." Find one that looks like you, put your initials on it, and fall in love all over again.

Fill It with Love

If it's going to be a long-term relationship, however, you're going to have to fill it with love, too. Okay, so you may not be putting your favorite Little Debbie cakes in there, but with a little planning and creativity, your lunch can still bring a smile. See the sample Ignite and Melt eating plans on pages 216–219 for suggestions on what to eat for your midday meals and snacks. Here is one possible combination that you could pack in your lunch box:

Lettuce wrap with turkey and fat-free cheese, spread with olive oil mayo

Sliced green and yellow peppers with hummus

Sugar-free pudding (for emergency chocolate cravings)

Sparkling water with lime

Almonds (for crunch!)

See, that doesn't sound so bad. And you don't have to reinvent the wheel every time. Make double portions at dinner so that you'll have enough left over to pack and reheat for lunch. Be sure to vary tastes and textures, and use the plan-approved seasonings below to give the food a little punch. Mix it up!

And take the time to pack your lunch the night before. I *know* this is easier said than done, but for the next few weeks, that little lunch box is a huge part of your diet. Give it priority and make sure it's packed with a plan-worthy lunch and snacks *before* the morning rush hits. Too much temptation happens if you head out the door without a lunch plan in your hand.

Do whatever it takes to make eating healthy a positive experience. (Remember, *so* much rides on your attitude.) Take a quick trip to your dollar store and buy some fun, colorful napkins, some plastic utensils and fun containers, and even ask hubby or the kids to pack a note for you, too. Silly? You (and they) won't think so when you're rocking a healthier, happier, skinnier new you.

Bam! Kick Up the Flavor!

Back in the dinosaur era, when I was doing fitness and figure competitions, everyone ate bland foods like flavorless chicken breasts and vegetables to drop weight and body fat quickly, and living on that stuff almost made me go crazy. I've since learned that there's no reason to deny yourself good flavor. You can still drop inches and body fat quickly with food that doesn't taste like paste. I want you to know what I wish someone had told *me* years ago: You can eat your chicken and have your flavor, too.

Thanks to the explosion of variety in herbs and spices on the shelves of most grocery stores, you can easily find a way to punch up the flavor of any breakfast, lunch, or dinner. There is no reason you can't cook a delicious dish that will leave you feeling totally satisfied. You will find a list of sensational seasonings and other flavor-blasted condiments in Chapter 6, but here are some tips on what to pair them with to truly make your meals sing!

CHEF JASON'S FLAVOR PROFILES

I've enlisted the help of one of Tennessee's top chefs, Jason McConnell, to help us out with flavor combos.

Here are some flavors that work very well together. Pick and choose within each list.

Asian: chile, lime, cilantro, soy, sesame oil, rice wine vinegar, ginger, garlic

Greek: olives, olive oil, red wine vinegar, dill, oregano, feta cheese, red-pepper flakes, mint

Indian: curry powder, cilantro, mint, yogurt, chiles, lemon, ginger, garlic

Italian: basil, oregano, thyme, olive oil, balsamic vinegar, red wine vinegar, garlic, parmesan

Mexican: cumin, coriander, chili powder, citrus, chiles, garlic, cilantro

Marinades:

Lemon, garlic, olive oil, basil, thyme

Soy, ginger, chili paste, sesame oil

Sugar-free jelly, Dijon mustard

Yogurt, curry powder, garlic, lemon, ground red pepper

Herbs (Fresh and Dried)

Basil lends a pungent Italian flavor to meat, poultry, fish, pasta, pizza, soup, or veggies.

Bay leaves add spice and fragrance to soups, stews, and veggies.

Cilantro gives meat, poultry, fish, rice, salads, and salsa a zesty southwestern kick.

Garlic adds smooth, buttery heat to meat, poultry, soups, sauces, marinades, and sautés—and makes them smell fantastic.

CHEF JASON'S FLAVOR 101

- Salt, salt, salt: Salt should be used in moderation, but it is a great flavor enhancer and can really take an okay dish to the next level. I generally use kosher salt because it has a larger grain than iodized salt and allows you better control. You can see and feel exactly how much you are using.

- You can replace salt with light soy sauce, hot sauce, or olives. All of these are concentrated with sodium and provide additional flavor. (Note: Consuming sodium in excessive amounts can lead to bloating, so use sodium-concentrated products in moderation.)

- When you're using herbs, the rule of thumb is 1 tablespoon dry = 3 tablespoons fresh.

- Vinegars have their place. You can use a robust vinegar (like balsamic) in your salad dressing and maybe a mild one (like rice wine) in a soup or marinade.

- Vinegars and citrus juices can really brighten a dish. A fresh lemon squeezed over the top of grilled fish or chicken really adds a ton of flavor.

- Mustards are great to use in marinades. They add a bit of spice and salt and will help fresh herbs adhere to the protein.

Oregano is very pungent, so use this sharp Italian herb in moderation on meat, poultry, fish, veggies, beans, pasta, and pizza.

Parsley adds a light, mild zest to poultry, fish, eggs, pasta, potatoes, rice, and veggies. Fresh parsley also makes a beautiful green garnish.

Sage brings a slightly bitter, minty taste to meat, poultry, fish, beans, and veggies. It also pairs well with cheese and, believe it or not, apples!

Thyme lends a pungent, minty, light-lemon aroma to meat, poultry, fish, veggies, soups, and potatoes. It also pairs wonderfully with goat cheese.

SPICES MADE SIMPLE

Buy premixed seasonings according to the type of food you're cooking. For example: Choose poultry seasoning if you're cooking chicken, lemon pepper for fish, Italian seasoning if you're making an Italian dish, Cajun or Creole spices for those dishes, and BBQ for grilling. Caution: These premixed seasons can be full of salt and sometimes sugar. Check the label!

Spices

Black peppercorns bring heat and a hint of sweetness to meat, poultry, fish, salads, soups, and eggs. They pair especially well with tomatoes and—for an unexpected, spicy dessert—strawberries.

Cumin adds an enticing Indian fragrance to meat, poultry, fish, soups, stews, beans, curries, couscous, and rice.

Lemon pepper lends an alluring combination of citrus and heat to chicken, fish, and veggies.

Paprika gives a light, subtle spiciness to meat, poultry, fish, shellfish, potatoes, and cauliflower.

Sauces, Vinegars, and Pastes

Balsamic vinegar is a tart, slightly sweet complement to steaks, salads, tomatoes, and strawberries. Mix it with olive oil for a light vinaigrette dressing.

Chicken, beef, or vegetable stock makes a hearty, savory base for soups, stews, purees, and sautéed vegetables.

Extra-virgin olive oil has a lemony, buttery flavor perfect for sautéing meat, poultry, and vegetables and drizzling on salad.

Tabasco sauce is a hot, spicy complement to any dish that needs a little heat! Try it on grilled chicken or eggs.

Tahini is a slightly bitter sesame seed paste used to make hummus that adds a tangy, Middle Eastern flair to soups and sauces.

Wasabi adds a sharp, very fiery zing to sushi and sashimi.

Worcestershire sauce makes a tart, savory base for meat and poultry sauces, marinades, and stir-fries.

Take It Outside

Let's face it: Exercising indoors can get a little monotonous, and it is very easy to get distracted with lingering laundry, clinging kids, and a constantly buzzing cell phone! No wonder it feels as if you can't find time to exercise. If you're champing at the bit and dying for a change of pace and scenery, take it outside. Fresh air, beautiful nature, open space—what's not to love?

As long as you're prepared, you can head out the door no matter what the season. Here are some precautions you should take—winter, summer, spring, or fall.

Exercising in the Heat

Drink. You need to stay hydrated before, during, and after exercising in the heat in order to replenish all the fluids you will lose through sweat. You should drink 7 to 10 ounces of water every 15 to 20 minutes. If you are going to be working out strenuously for a long period of time, you will also need to replace your electrolytes with a low-sugar sports drink like EcoDrink or G2* to help avoid heatstroke or heat exhaustion.

---

*EcoDrink is a sugar-free, calorie-free drink that claims to hydrate and be five times better for you than leading vitamin waters. It contains 31 vitamins and minerals. G2 is the lighter version of Gatorade (it has 20 calories and 5 grams of sugar per serving).

Chill. Take it easier than you would if you were working out in an air-conditioned room. Your body needs to become acclimated to the heat. If you are used to exercising in cold weather or a cool gym, don't go for a 5-mile run at noon on your beach vacation. Do a little each day until your body gets used to the weather.

Dress the part. Be sure to wear light-colored clothing so that it will reflect the sun. Also, this is not the time to be shy and dress in layers. Girl, let it all hang out! The hotter it is outside, the less you should have on. Your clothes should also be loose fitting and made of moisture-wicking materials to keep you cool. Don't forget your sunblock!

Change time. My personal rule of thumb is, if it's 90 degrees or higher, don't risk breaking a sweat outside and getting yourself sick. You can avoid the heat of the day by working out early in the morning or later in the evening as the sun is going down. This is also true for humidity. In general, if you start to feel dizzy or nauseated during your workout, stop and get out of the heat.

Exercising in the Cold

When temperatures fall, you need to be very aware of hypothermia, a life-threatening condition in which your body loses too much of its heat to function properly. Hypothermia is just as dangerous as heat exhaustion or heatstroke, so make sure you are prepared to safely hit the ground running in winter weather. My policy: If it's below 42 degrees, I'm staying indoors. I see crazy people running in 20-degree weather, but I don't think the reward is worth the risk of serious illness or injury from slipping on ice or snow. When in doubt, don't go out.

Dress the part. Now is the time to put on the layers. You need to isolate your body heat so it doesn't escape. Wear moisture-wicking clothing that will trap the air but still allow sweat to pass through.

Cover your digits. When the weather gets cold, it can cause blood to move away from your hands and feet to the center of your body in order to keep your ticker and other vital parts working properly. This blood flow can cause damage to your extremities, so put on gloves and wear thick socks under your sneakers.

Cover your melon. You can lose up to 80 percent of your body heat through your head, and nothing hurts worse than frozen ears! Wear a fitted hat or cap that won't fall off or down onto your eyes while you are exercising.

Supercharge My Skinny

Jump! Jump!

Jumping rope is a wonderful exercise. It's convenient, it's easy, and it's one major calorie-blasting workout. In only 15 minutes of skipping rope, you can burn 160 calories! So when the weather is bad or you've run out of time to go to the gym, go home, put on some high-energy music, and get hopping. If you (or your kids) don't have a jump rope already, you can buy one super cheap at a toy or discount store. They're also light and easy to pack for a quick workout on the road.

If the rope trips you up or you're caught somewhere without one, jump without it! Perform the arm motions as if you're turning the rope while jumping or skipping around the room. You can even get fancy (with or *without* the rope), switching feet, crossing arms, or "skiing" from side to side as you jump.

Jumping rope is the ultimate excuse buster. You don't need a gym. You don't need fancy equipment. You just need to *jump!*

The Scale Is a Hormonal B—ch

That seemingly innocent scale in your bathroom can really mess with your emotions—and destroy your confidence. One day she'll show you a fabulous number, and you can almost hear her saying, "Did you lose weight?"

Then, when you least expect it (like the very next day)—*wham!*—she stabs you in the back with some way-higher digits.

You have to arm yourself against her.

How do you do that, you ask? Don't give her the power.

And how do you do that? You stay away from her. She can't get to you if you don't get on her. *Period!*

Why She's So Emotional

Ruthless as she is, the scale does have a lot of factors that can affect her mood.

1. Time of day. Unlike me, the scale is much nicer in the mornings. This is mainly because you haven't eaten anything in the last 8 hours or so. As the day goes on you will weigh more, depending on how much food and liquid you have in your stomach. If you want to see your lowest weight, get on the scale first thing in the morning with nothing on, before eating and after using the bathroom.

2. Salt and water. Salt retains water. Water flushes salt. Salt: bad. Water: good. Processed foods are outlawed on this plan because of the amount of salt they contain. If you drink plenty of water, you'll flush out the salt, and your body won't feel the need to store excess water because it's getting plenty. Drink it up, baby!

3. Time of the month. Of course, when the curse comes a-calling, you're going to blow up like the Goodyear Blimp, and yep, you guessed it: You're going to weigh more. As many as 4 pounds more. If you have your period or are just about to start it, don't go anywhere near the scale.

Skinny Fiction: A Calorie Is a Calorie?

Well, yes and no. Yes, 100 calories is just that—100 calories—but not all calories are created equal. If that were the case, you could eat 1,500 calories of nothing but Dove chocolates every day and have a stealth body. Oh, don't I wish that were the case! But, as we've discussed, your body doesn't like having its insulin spiked. Think of it this way: A healthy fiber- or protein-packed 100 calories is like a luxurious car that makes you look sexy when you pull up for a night out with the girls. A fatty, salty, sugary 100 calories is a jalopy that needs a new paint job and you can't breathe because of the black plume of smoke coming from the exhaust. Which do you want to roll?

4. Body composition. If you are working this plan 100 percent, the scale may not move a whole lot after the first couple of weeks. Why? Because you are changing your body composition. This is a good thing! You are replacing the fluffy fat weight with lean muscle weight. They may weigh the same, but muscle takes up much less room, and you will look slimmer and more toned. See "Skinny Fiction: Muscle Weighs More Than Fat" on page 186.

> **SKINNY 411**
> Your body uses 45 different muscles to take one step. *Keep taking steps!*

5. Dirty pipes. You will weigh more or less depending on how much rubbish you have in your intestines. Of course there's the day-to-day digestion that goes on. It takes about 4 hours to digest most foods. But there's also a gross little factoid that most people don't consider. Over the years, your intestines can store a gunky buildup, much like the pipes going out of your house. The average person can have 5 to 40 pounds of built-up fecal matter in her colon.[2] This buildup will show on the scale, too! Someone say, "Ew!"

Size Matters

We are women. Our weight is constantly fluctuating—sometimes up to 5 pounds in a single day. So don't be a slave to the scale. It's not your weight that matters; it's how well your clothes fit. Let your skinny jeans be your guide.

Want to see the numbers that do matter? Follow the instructions starting below to measure yourself at the end of each week and record your measurements in the spaces provided. You'll be thrilled to see how much you are shrinking!

1. Grab a tape measure.

2. Wearing just your underwear, pull the tape measure around your chest (not your arms) and measure at the fullest point.

3. Measure the circumference of the largest part of both your left and right upper arms.

4. Measure the circumference of your waist at the smallest point, just above your navel.

5. Measure the circumference of your hips at the widest point. This is usually the vertical center point of your butt.

6. Measure the circumference of each of your thighs about midway between the hip and the knee.

Chest: _____ inches

Upper Arm: L _____ inches R _____ inches

Waist: _____ inches

Hips: _____ inches

Thigh: L _____ inches R _____ inches

Become a Master Mind

"All personal breakthroughs begin with a change in beliefs."
—Anthony Robbins

Yes, I'm gonna say it again. If you're not 100 percent committed to yourself, you might as well use this book as a coaster. Don't roll your eyes at me!

Remember DEA? You've got to get it down. You've got to eat, sleep, and breathe it. Take control of your thoughts and actions. If you don't, they *will* take control of you.

Homework!

What *don't* you like about your current body?

_____

_____

_____

What *do* you like about your current body?

_____

_____

_____

Did you have any fears or apprehension about doing this program? If so, why do you think you are scared? _____

_____

_____

_____

What can you do today to shut up any negative voices in your head?

_____

_____

_____

Who are your biggest supporters?

_____

_____

_____

Who is your biggest saboteur or hater?

_____

_____

_____

THE SKINNY—*From Someone Who's Been There*

"It was amazing; all of my cravings disappeared after the first week!"
—*Leah, Skinny Jeans Rock Star (page 54)*

What's Your Excuse?

Let's face it: Excuses are like exes. We've all got (at least) one. You may have a whole list of them, and if you don't nip them in the bud, you could be weaseling your way out of ever seeing those skinny jeans. How do you prevent that from happening? First, acknowledge that you are making excuses, and then work on changing them one by one.

Use the spaces below to spill all your excuses, and next to each one, write out how you *can* actually do what you are trying to get out of. If you're perfect and don't have any excuses, congratulations. Write something anyway—maybe a little love note to yourself. I've started you off with my two biggest excuses.

Why I Can't . . .

I don't have time to exercise.
I hate to cook!

_____

_____

_____

_____

How I Can!

I will schedule time for myself.
I will find something about cooking that I enjoy.

_____

_____

_____

_____

My Skinny Check-In

☐ I tried some new flavor combinations.

☐ I tracked my diet and exercise every day.

☐ I found a workout buddy!

☐ I Supercharged My Skinny!

☐ I completed this week's attitude homework.

☐ I kept a great attitude!

☐ I worked the plan! I worked the plan! I worked the plan!

Skinny Jeans
ROCK ST★R

Before: Size 8   After: Size 6

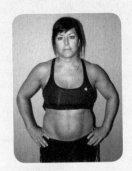

Name: Carey

Age: 42

Occupation: Entertainment manager and producer

Children: 2

Pounds lost: 17.7

What I was afraid of: Failing myself. Could I, would I, stick with it? I will miss my wine.

What I liked: I loved the workouts—and the best part was, I could do them from home. Sometimes my family did them with me!

What I learned: I have willpower and strength. Having a regimen and a strong program to work makes all the difference. And there is life without wine!

What I want to share: I used to say that I wanted to be a smoking-hot mom. But I'm not looking to be the object of desire by other men. I wanted to fall in love with me again. Of course, it's nice to have my husband's attention, too.

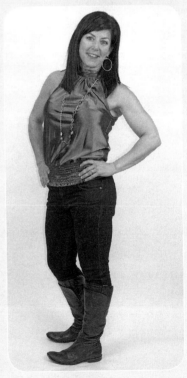

Chapter 5

THE WORKOUTS

It's time to move it, shake it, and slap it into shape! Yeah, baby!

I hope you are as excited as I am! Now, I'm not going to lie to you; when done as prescribed, these workouts are hard, but they are *fun,* and they *work!* None of them requires big, fancy exercise equipment or a health club membership. However, if you do want to add a little extra zing to your workouts, you can purchase a small set of dumbbells (about $15 per set), a resistance band (as low as $9), and a yoga-style mat for the Blast workout (about $18). You can also find *Six Weeks to Skinny Jeans* workout kits at www.amycotta.com

Last-Minute Details

Be careful when you exercise with resistance bands. Always check the band for fraying or tears. If you find a tear, don't use the band! It can snap and potentially injure you. To extend the life of your band, use it only on smooth surfaces. Rough flooring or pavement will cause the rubber to break down and rip faster.

There are four ways to adjust the resistance of your band. If you stand on it with only one foot, it will be at its lightest tension. Standing with both feet will make the resistance harder. If you need even more resistance while doing bicep curls, stand with both feet at the center point of the band and crisscross the handles, forming an X. This will make the exercise even harder. You can also make the band harder by taking up some of the slack. For example, if you want to add resistance to your squats without having to hold the handles up by your shoulders, stand on the band with your hands at your sides and wrap it around your hands until you reach the desired resistance.

You can't adjust the weight of a traditional dumbbell, but you can make it harder to use. Slow down the tempo of the entire movement, thus increasing the burn. Or do what is called a negative rep. Here's an example: Use a normal tempo on the way up to the top of the movement. Once you reach the top, lower the weight super slowly (use a count of 10 to 20 to complete the rep). Once you're at the starting point of the exercise, repeat.

Don't forget to start each workout with a proper warmup.

Okay. Are you ready? Let's get this party started.

The Warmup

WHAT YOU NEED

An open space

A sturdy chair (optional for balance)

What you need to know: You should do this warmup routine every day before performing any of the workouts. Do 1 set of 8 to 10 reps of each exercise. If you are using one leg at a time, perform 8 to 10 reps on each leg. This warmup will help prevent injuries and offset muscle soreness. If you'd like, you can also do this warmup for your cooldown/stretch in addition to The Daily Lube (see page 112). To see video clips of these exercises, visit www.amycotta.com.

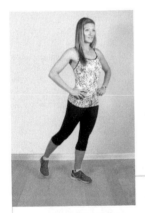 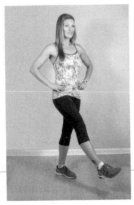 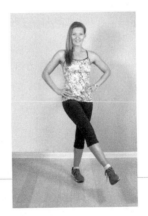 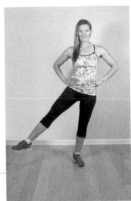

LEG SWINGS

Stand (holding on to the back of the chair if you are using one), allowing your right leg to hang loosely, without tension. Swing this leg front to back, allowing the muscle to stretch through the motion. After 8 to 10 reps, take the leg out to the side and let it swing in front of your body, crossing its midline, then back to the side. Repeat front and side swings on your left leg.

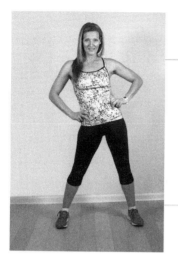

HIP CIRCLES

Stand with your feet about hip width apart and place your hands on your hips. Move your hips slowly to the right, then complete a full circle back to the front. Once you've completed 8 to 10 circles in this direction, continue circling for 8 to 10 reps in the opposite direction.

KNEE CIRCLES

Stand with your legs and feet together. Bend at the knees, placing your hands above your knees on your thighs. Keeping your legs together, make circles with your knees and your ankles. Complete 8 to 10 reps in both directions.

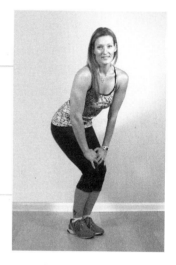

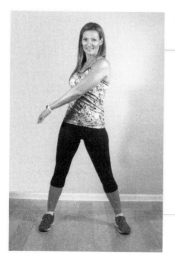

TWISTS

Stand with your feet shoulder width apart. Allow your arms to dangle at your sides. Your upper body should be free of all tension. From the waist, twist your upper body from right to left. Your arms should still be dangling, but the twisting movement will make them move slightly from side to side. Be sure to keep your shoulders relaxed down and away from your ears. Do 8 to 10 reps.

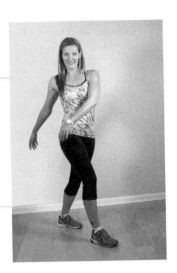

TWISTS WITH ONE LEG OUT FRONT

Stand in a staggered position with your knees bent and your right foot in front. Keeping your hips forward, perform the same twisting movement as the above exercise. Do 8 to 10 reps and then repeat with your left leg forward.

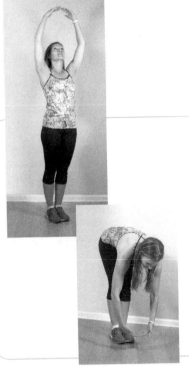

SWAN DIVES

Stand up straight with your feet close together and your knees slightly bent. Raise your arms above your head and bend down from the waist. Sweep your hands down toward the ground as if trying to pick something up. Then, with your fingertips touching, raise your hands out in front of you and slowly raise your torso back up so that you are standing tall again. Once your arms are over your head, open up your chest and press your hips forward. Return to your beginning position and repeat for 8 to 10 reps.

Blast Workout

WHAT YOU NEED

An open space

Comfortable workout clothes and sneakers

A set of dumbbells (5 to 10 pounds) and/or a light-to-medium resistance band

Water

What you need to know: Perform the Blast exercises in the sequence in which they are written, and complete all of the reps for each exercise before moving on to the next. As you will see in the chart below, you will increase the number of reps throughout the 6 weeks: performing 1 or 2 sets of 10, then 12, then 15. Any exercise that is listed as "alternating" will be performed on both sides to count as 1 repetition. As you go through the Blast Workout, your legs should begin to feel tight and tired. To personalize your workout to your fitness level, see the "Too Hard?" and "Too Easy?" charts after each exercise. Also use the RPE Scale on page 22 to make sure you're working between 6 and 8, and adjust your workout accordingly. Watch video clips of the Blast Workout exercises at www.amycotta.com.

THE ROUTINE

WEEKS	SETS	REPS	REST
1 and 2	1 or 2	10	0–30 seconds
3 and 4	1 or 2	12	0–30 seconds
5 and 6	1 or 2	15	0–30 seconds

THE EXERCISES

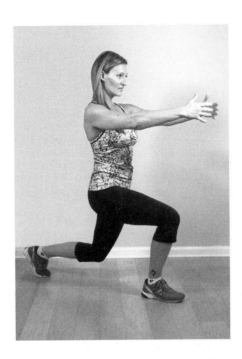 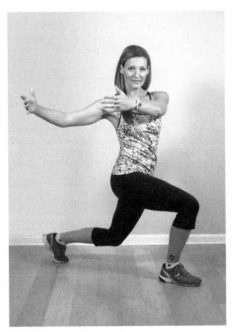

ALTERNATING FORWARD LUNGE WITH A TWIST

Stand with your feet about hip width apart and your arms stretched out in front of you, parallel to the floor. Lunge forward with your right foot, allowing your front and back knees to bend. Once you're in the lunge, keep your hips straight and facing forward, and then, twisting from your trunk, turn your arms and chest as far toward your front knee as your body will comfortably allow. Return your arms and upper body back to the straight-and-forward position. Push off the front leg to return to a standing position. Repeat with your left leg forward.

Too Hard?	*Too Easy?*
Start with a forward lunge without the twist. Once your balance improves, you can add the twist.	Try going lower into the lunge, or hold dumbbells while you perform the twists.

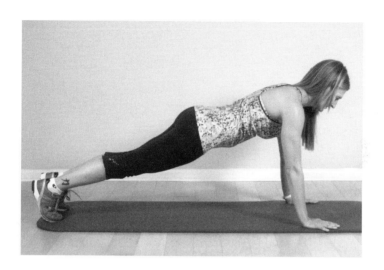

PUSHUPS

Start in a plank position on either your knees or toes. Place your hands out from your chest more than shoulder width apart. Be sure to keep your spine in a straight line. Slowly lower your chest to the ground, then raise back up to the starting position.

Too Hard?

Perform the pushups on your knees.

Too Easy?

Perform the pushups on your toes. Complete the motion very slowly.

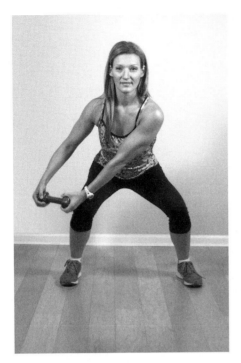 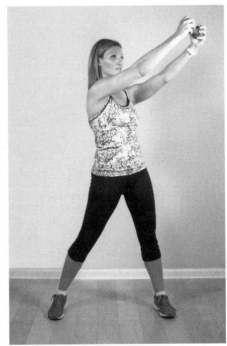

WOOD CHOPS

Stand with your feet about hip to shoulder width apart. Squat down while keeping your chest raised, eyes straight ahead. As you squat, reach both arms down to your right side, twisting slightly at the waist. As you rise up out of the squat, raise your arms in a diagonal motion toward the left side of your body and up over your head. Keep your abs tight, because the twisting motion will work your entire core. Complete reps and then repeat on the other side.

Too Hard?

Keep your squat shallow.

Too Easy?

Take your squat deeper.

Hold a dumbbell or use a resistance band.

If you're using a resistance band, lay it on the ground, stand on it with both feet, and hold the handle with both hands. There should be enough slack in the band to perform the exercise without limitation.

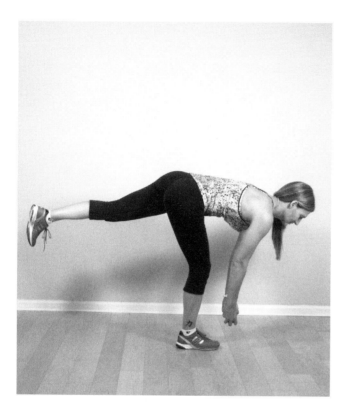
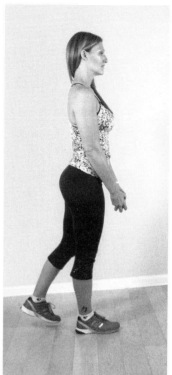

SINGLE-LEG DEAD LIFTS

Stand on one foot with your base knee slightly bent. Keeping your hips and shoulders squared and your chest open, abs tight, slowly bend forward from your torso, and reach down toward your toes. As you bend forward, your back leg will lift upward. Tighten your glutes and slowly rise up and repeat. Complete all of your reps on one side before moving on to the next.

Too Hard?

Do the same movement but keep both legs on the floor. Or use a single leg, but allow your back foot to touch the floor for balance.

Too Easy?

Hold the dumbbells in your hands. Keep your back leg perfectly straight as you lift it. Slow down the movement.

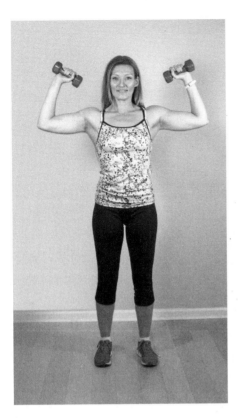
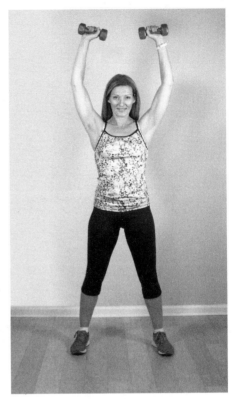

SHOULDER PRESS

Stand holding one dumbbell in each hand or a resistance band at your shoulders, palms facing out. Slowly push the dumbbells or band up toward the ceiling, stopping just before your arms are fully extended. Return to your shoulders and repeat.

Too Hard?

Use lighter dumbbells. Alternate arms, pushing them up one at a time instead of together.

Too Easy?

Use heavier dumbbells. Try a harder version of the resistance band. Perform the motion very slowly.

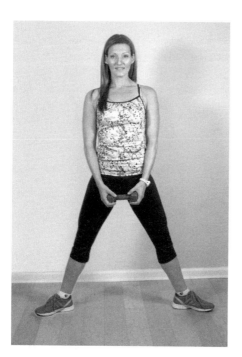 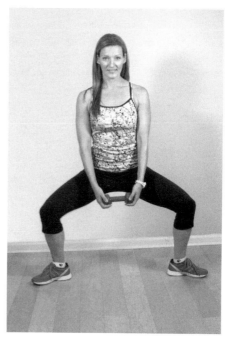

PLIÉ SQUAT

Stand up straight with your feet wider than shoulder width apart and turn your feet slightly so that your toes are pointing outward. (Only turn them out as far as it is comfortable. If you took ballet as a kid, getting into a plié position should be easy.) Be sure to keep your pelvis tucked so that your behind is not sticking out. Think about keeping your upper body and core as straight as a board. (You can hold a dumbbell as shown, but it is not required.) Lower yourself into a squat with your knees pointing out to each side. Only go as far down as your body will comfortably allow. As you start to move back up, squeeze your glutes and push your weight through your feet as if you're trying to push them through the floor. Straighten your legs until your knees are just shy of being locked.

Too Hard?	*Too Easy?*
Don't go down as far.	Take the squat lower.
	Hold a dumbbell at your pelvis.
	Hold two dumbbells at your shoulders.
	Pause at the bottom of the move.

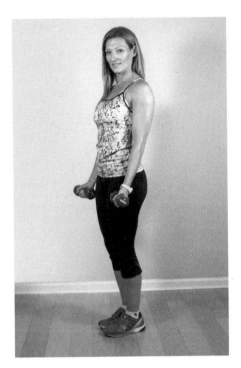
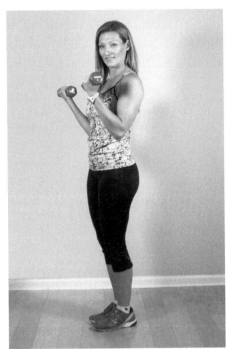

BICEPS CURLS

Hold your arms down at your sides with either dumbbells or a resistance band in each hand. Keep your arms glued to your sides and slowly bend up at the elbow, contracting your biceps and turning your palms in toward your body as you draw your hands toward your shoulders. Lower your hands and repeat.

Too Hard?	*Too Easy?*
Use a lighter weight (a 16-oz bottle of water would work) or resistance band.	Use a heavier dumbbell, harder resistance band stance, or negative reps. If you don't have anything heavier, perform the reps super slowly—really concentrating on the muscle contraction.

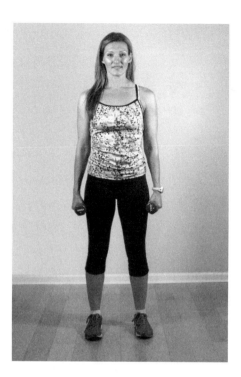
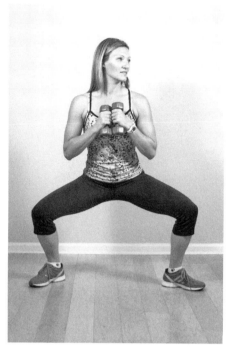

DROP STEPS

Stand with your feet hip width apart. Step back with your right foot and then extend it out to your right about 90 degrees. This starting position resembles a martial arts fighting stance. Perform a squat, going as deep as your body will allow and keeping your weight evenly distributed on both legs. Shift your weight to your front leg as you push off the floor. Rise out of the squat and return the right foot to its starting position. Perform all reps with your right leg back and then repeat with your left leg back.

Too Hard?	*Too Easy?*
Keep the squat portion of the move shallow.	Go lower into the move.
	Hold dumbbells in front of your chest or at your shoulders.
	Take a pause at the bottom of the squat.

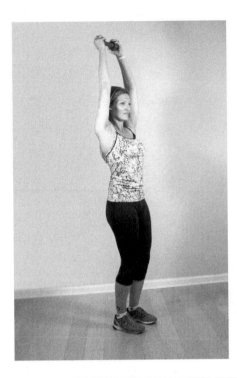
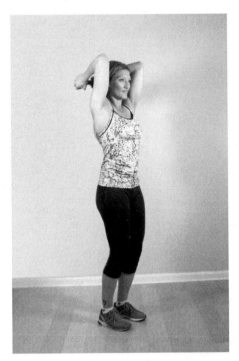

TRICEPS EXTENSIONS

Stand tall with your feet shoulder width apart. Holding a dumbbell with an end in either hand, pull your arms up by your ears and lock them into place. Your arms should be straight and fully extended upward. Without moving your shoulders, bend your elbows, allowing the dumbbells to drop toward your back. Raise the dumbbells back above your head and repeat.

Too Hard?

Use lighter dumbbells.

Too Easy?

Use heavier dumbbells.

Perform the movement very slowly.

Use a resistance band: Place the band on the ground, step on it with your right foot, and put your left foot forward so that you are in a staggered stance.

Hold the handles up by your ears and bend your elbows so that they drop toward your back.

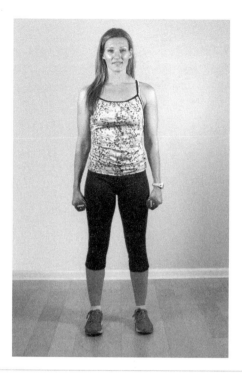
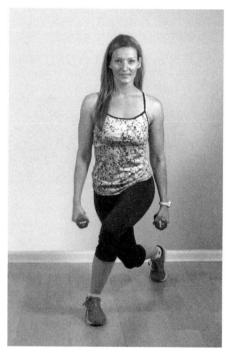

ALTERNATING CURTSY LUNGES

Stand with your feet about hip width apart, a dumbbell in either hand. Keep your left leg in place and lunge backward, crossing your right leg behind your left one. Most of your weight should be on your left foot while you rest on the ball of your right foot and use it like a kickstand for balance. Slowly lower yourself so that both knees bend. Keep your chest up, your back straight, and your hips squared. At the bottom of the movement, you should be curtsying as if you were meeting the queen. Push your weight up off of the front foot, bringing your right foot back to its starting position. Repeat with your left leg back.

Too Hard?	*Too Easy?*
Don't lunge as deeply, or do a regular lunge with your leg going directly behind you instead of over to the side.	Take the lunge lower.
	Pause at the bottom of the movement.
	Bring your lunging leg up into a high front knee before going back into the curtsy.
	Hold heavier dumbbells at your side as you curtsy.

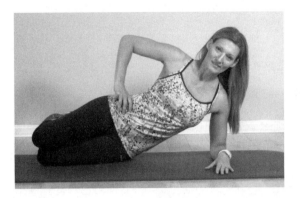

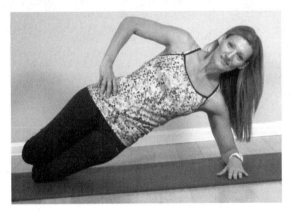

SIDE PLANK CRUNCH

Lie on your left side with your knees bent. Bend your bottom elbow to 90 degrees so that it's in an L shape, with your fingers pointing away from your body and your elbow directly under your shoulder, supporting your torso. Be sure to keep your joints stacked: Your ankles, knees, and hips should be lined up on top of one another. Slowly raise your bottom hip off the ground. Initiate the movement from the oblique (side abdominal muscle) that's closest to the ground. Squeeze at the top of the movement. Slowly return your hip to the floor. Complete all reps on your left side before repeating on your right.

Too Hard?	*Too Easy?*
Hold the plank and skip the crunch.	Instead of resting on your knees, straighten out your legs and do the crunches using the side of your bottom foot as your base.

Firm Workout

WHAT YOU NEED

An open space

Comfortable workout clothes (sneakers are optional)

Plenty of water

A clock or watch with a second hand (optional)

A yoga-style mat (optional)

What you need to know: This workout is based on the slow-burn principle. In other words, you will be moving v-e-r-y s-l-o-w-l-y! Each repetition will last for a count of 10 or for 10 seconds on the clock (5 seconds up, 5 seconds down). Use a clock or watch to time yourself, or just count in your head. You will perform reps of all the exercises on the right side of your body *before* going back and performing the same number of reps of each exercise on the left. If your legs feel as if they're on fire, you're doing it right! If you need to take a quick stretch in between exercises, go ahead, but you *need* to perform them in the sequence listed here. If you want an added challenge, feel free to add a resistance band loop: a small circular band that you can place around your ankles or thighs and hold for added tension. They come in light, medium, and heavy resistance.

THE ROUTINE

WEEKS	SETS	REPS	TIME/COUNT
1 and 2	1 or 2	5 (each side)	10 seconds
3 and 4	1 or 2	8 (each side)	10 seconds
5 and 6	1 or 2	10 (each side)	10 seconds

THE EXERCISES

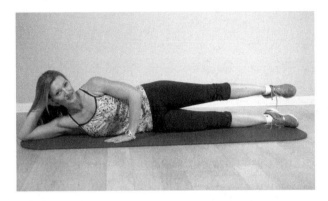

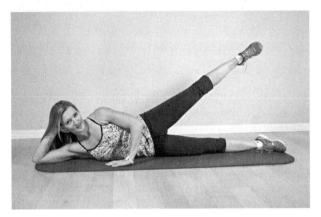

SIDE LEG LIFTS

Lie on your side with your body in a straight line, keeping your joints stacked. Your top leg should hover just above the bottom one, but the legs shouldn't touch. While squeezing your glutes (butt muscles), slowly raise your leg until your foot is about 45 degrees from your hip. Slowly lower your leg.

Too Hard?	*Too Easy?*
Pause and shake out your leg when needed.	Go slower.
	Squeeze your glutes harder.
	Add a resistance loop around your thighs.

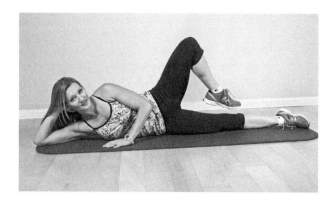

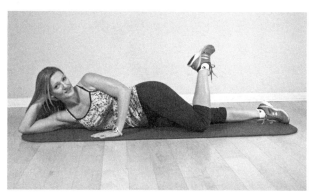

KNEE TOES

Lie on your side in a straight line, keeping your joints stacked. Bend the knee of your top leg so that it's pointing toward the sky. Place the toe of your top leg on the knee of your bottom leg. While maintaining your body position, slowly rotate at the hip so that the top knee moves toward the floor and foot toward the sky. Squeeze your glutes and return the knee to its upward starting position.

Too Hard?	*Too Easy?*
Pause and shake it out when needed.	Go slower.
	Squeeze your glutes harder.
	Add a resistance loop around your thighs.

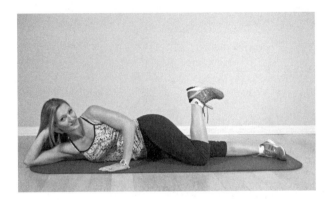

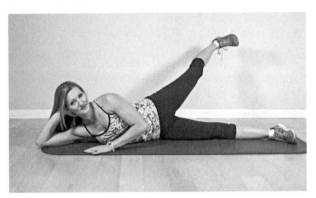

LYING DONKEY KICK

Lie on your side in a straight line, keeping your joints stacked. Pull your top knee in toward your chest and angle it toward the ground. Your hip will rotate slightly toward the ground as well. Flex your top foot and slowly drive it back behind you at about a 45-degree angle (squeezing your glutes the whole way). Draw the knee back in toward the starting position and repeat.

Too Hard?	*Too Easy?*
Pause and shake it out when needed.	Go slower. Squeeze harder!
	Add a resistance band around your thighs.

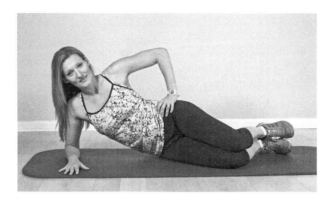

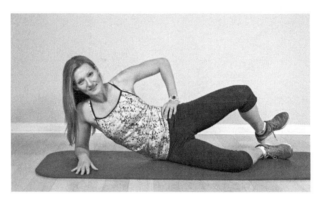

CLAMSHELL

Lie on your side with your joints stacked. Pull your knees in toward your chest at a 45-degree angle from your hip. Squeeze your abs and your glutes, and keeping your heels together, slowly separate your knees and toes. Open as far as you can without your heels coming apart.

Too Hard?	*Too Easy?*
Pause and shake it out when needed.	Go slower.
	Squeeze your abs and glutes harder.
	Add a resistance loop around your thighs.

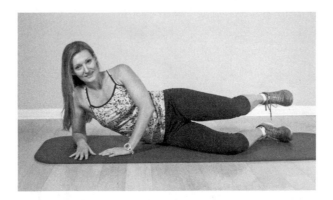

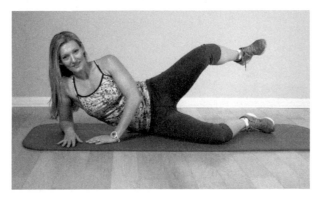

OPEN THE DOOR

Lie in the same body position as the clamshell exercise you just performed, with your joints stacked and your knees drawn up. Squeeze your glutes and slowly raise your top leg, with your knees, heels, and toes all coming apart from your bottom leg. (It's like a side leg lift but with bent knees.) Lift as high as you can without losing your body positioning. Then slowly lower.

Too Hard?	*Too Easy?*
Pause and shake it out when needed.	Go slower.
	Squeeze your abs and glutes harder.
	Add a resistance loop around your thighs.

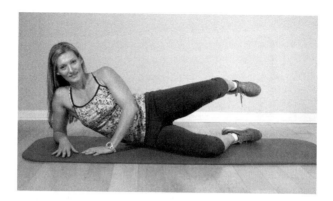

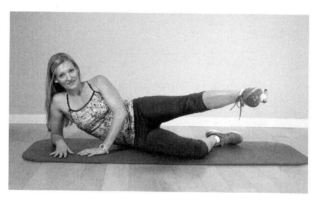

ISOLATED FRONT KICK

Keeping the same body positioning as the previous Open the Door exercise, raise your top leg until it's about 10 inches above your bottom leg. Keep your hip still and use your knee like a hinge to bring your heel toward your behind. Keeping the rest of your body still, slowly bring your foot forward until the knee is fully extended.

Too Hard?	*Too Easy?*
Pause and shake it out when needed.	Go slower.
	Squeeze your abs and glutes harder.
	Add a resistance loop around your thighs.

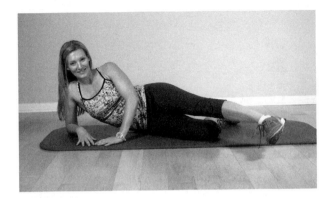

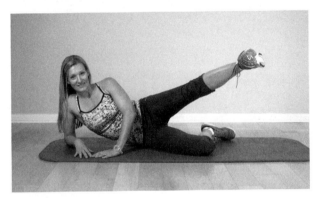

ISOLATED BOOTY BURNER

Keeping the same body position as in the Isolated Front Kick exercise, extend your top leg as straight out as possible without locking it. Keeping this leg hovering above your bottom leg, lift it as high as you comfortably can. Slowly return to the hovering position. Perform all reps on this side before switching to the other side.

Too Hard?	*Too Easy?*
Pause and shake it out when needed.	Go slower.
	Squeeze your abs and glutes harder.
	Add a resistance loop around your thighs.

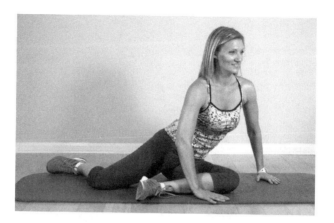

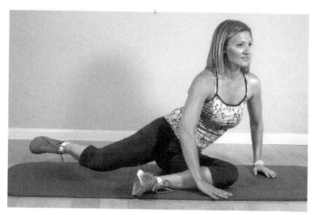

S LIFTS

Sit on the floor with your legs separated into an S shape: Each knee should be in a 90-degree angle, with the resting leg in the front and the working leg in the back. Place the hand of the nonworking side on the floor next to your leg. Bend forward slightly, with your chest lifted up, and lift your back leg up (while squeezing your glutes) about an inch off the floor. Perform all reps with this leg before switching to the other.

Too Hard?

Lean farther into the front leg.

Too Easy?

Go slower.

Squeeze your glutes harder!

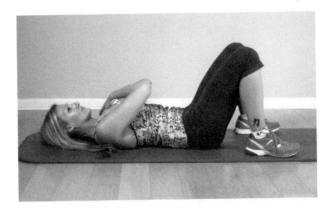

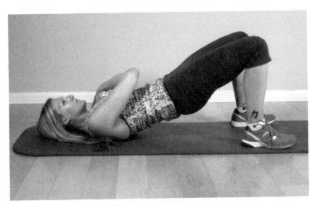

GLUTE RAISES

Lie flat on your back with your arms across your chest, your knees bent, and your feet flat on the ground. (You should look as if you're about to do crunches.) Slowly squeeze your glutes and raise your hips off the ground, lifting them as high as you can without lifting your shoulder blades off the floor. Slowly return to the starting position and repeat.

Too Hard?	*Too Easy?*
Don't raise your hips as high off the floor.	Lift your hips higher.
Place your hands at your side on the ground.	Squeeze your glutes harder.
	Hold dumbbells on your hip flexors (across your hips) so that you are lifting more weight.
	Add a resistance band around your thighs.

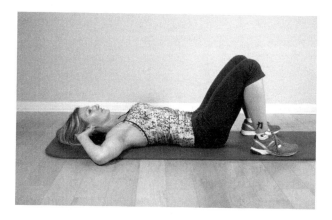

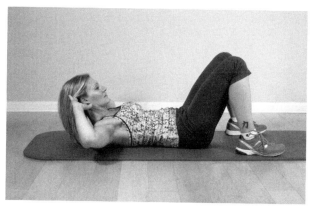

CRUNCHES

Lie flat on your back with your spine pressed into the floor. Place your feet on the floor with your knees bent, and hold your fingertips at your ears with your elbows bent. Start the contraction from your abdomen and slowly raise your shoulders off the ground. Exhale as you reach the top of the contraction (the tops of your shoulders should be off the floor). Slowly return and inhale on the way down.

Too Hard?	*Too Easy?*
Come on . . . really? They're just crunches.	Go slower on the up and down movements.
	Squeeze harder!
	Add a resistance band above your knees to keep your hips engaged.

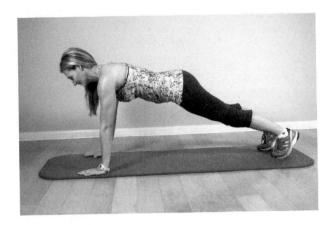

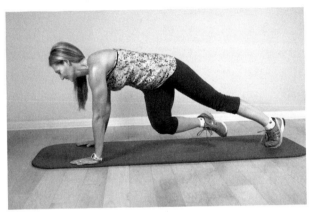

PRETZELS

Start in a plank pushup position. Be sure to keep your bottom down so that your back is almost flat. While squeezing your abs, pull your right knee in toward your chest and rotate it to your left shoulder. Then return it to the starting position. Repeat with your left leg. You will count each leg as 1 repetition.

Too Hard?	*Too Easy?*
Take out the twist and hold a regular plank.	Go slower.
	Squeeze your abs harder.
	Add a pushup in between each rep.

Burn Workout

WHAT YOU NEED

An open space

Comfortable workout clothes and sneakers

A clock or watch with a second hand

Plenty of water

What you need to know: Unless you need to take a break, you should move seamlessly from one exercise into the next. This workout will boost your heart rate and keep it up. You will increase your interval time throughout the 6 weeks, moving from 30 seconds to 45 seconds to 1 minute. Be sure to use the RPE Scale to keep yourself between 6 and 8. If you start to go above 8, take a break until your heart rate settles into a steadier yet still hardworking zone. You can watch video clips of Burn Workout exercises at www.amycotta.com.

THE ROUTINE

WEEKS	SETS	INTERVAL TIME	REST
1 and 2	1 or 2	30 seconds	0–60 seconds
3 and 4	1 or 2	45 seconds	0–30 seconds
5 and 6	1 or 2	1 minute	0–30 seconds

THE EXERCISES

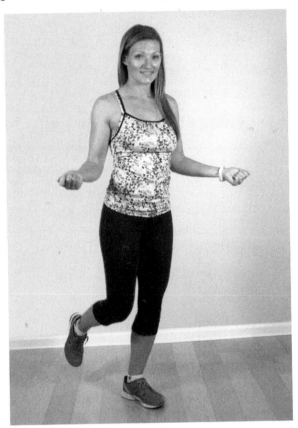

MOCK JUMP ROPE

Stand with your feet about hip width apart and hold your arms at your sides as though you were actually holding a jump rope. Jump lightly on the balls of your feet, mimicking real jump roping.

Too Hard?	*Too Easy?*
March in place.	Put more bounce in your step.
	Swing your arms in big circles.
	Add an actual jump rope!

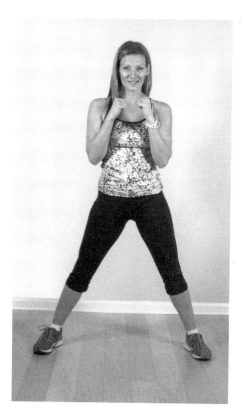 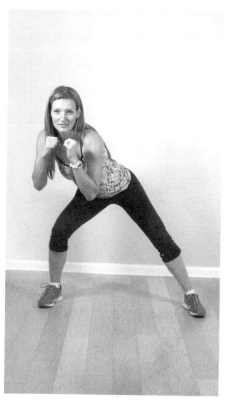

BOB AND WEAVE

Stand with your feet more than shoulder width apart. Sink down into a comfortable squat position. Now weave your upper body over to the right and rise up slightly out of the squat. Then lower yourself back into the squat position, weave over to the left, and back up out of the squat. Continue this motion, going from right to left and left to right. You will be mimicking ducking under something.

Too Hard?	*Too Easy?*
Keep the squat shallow. Perform the weave without the bob.	Take the squat deeper.
	Move faster.
	Punch out with your arms as you rise up on either side.

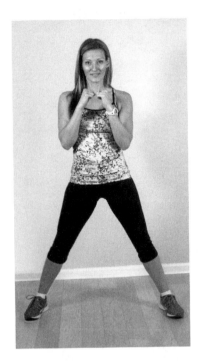
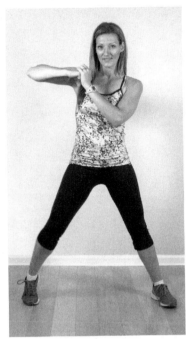
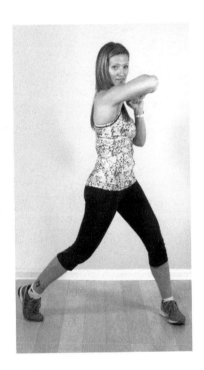

ELBOW STRIKES

Stand with your feet about shoulder width apart. Hold your hands in fists between your chest and chin, elbows bent and tucked toward your sides. Bend your right knee so that you are on the ball of your foot and raise your right elbow out to the side, keeping your fist at chin height. In one motion, rotate your right hip, leg, arm, and upper body to the left. Your elbow should completely cross your body, and your chest should be facing your left side. Return to your starting position and repeat on the other side. Keep alternating.

Too Hard?	*Too Easy?*
Come on . . . ?	Pick up the pace!

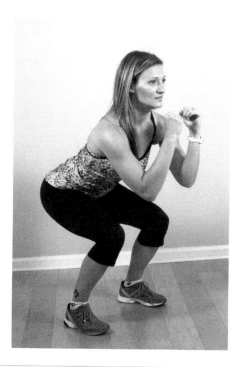
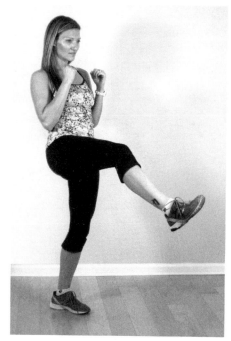

SQUATS WITH ALTERNATING SNAP KICKS

Stand with your feet about shoulder width apart. Perform a regular squat. As you rise out of the squat, lift your right knee and extend the foot forward in a kick. Retract your foot and place it back on the floor. Squat again, repeating the kick with your left leg. Keep alternating between squats with a right-leg kick and then with a left-leg kick.

Too Hard?

Keep your kicks low.

Keep squats shallow.

Too Easy?

Take squats deeper.

Take your kicks higher.

Take a small pause, or pulse up and down at the bottom of the squat.

Move faster.

Add a double fist punch with each kick.

Hold dumbbells at your shoulders or let them hang at your side.

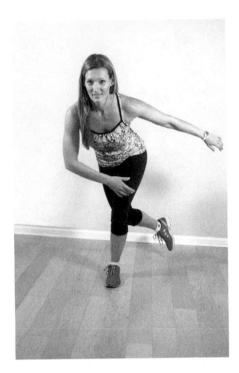
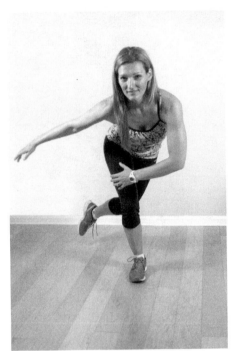

SPEED SKATERS

Stand with your feet hip width apart. Take a giant leap to your right side, landing on your right foot, keeping your knee soft and slightly bent as you land to absorb the impact. Let your left foot retract behind your right leg as if to lightly kick yourself in the behind. Your arms should swing out to the side as you jump from side to side. Now leap back to your left, landing on your left leg and bringing your right foot to the rear. Keep repeating and alternating sides. Think Olympic speed skating champion Apolo Anton Ohno.

Too Hard?	*Too Easy?*
Take out the hop and just take large steps from side to side. Don't use your arms.	Put a little more bounce in your step.
	Move faster.
	Go lower into the squat as you land on either side.

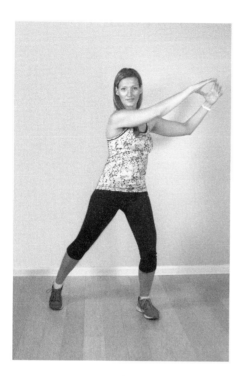 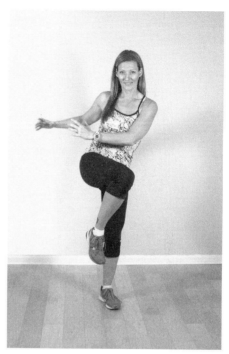

KNEE SMASHES

Start your stance with your left foot (which will be your base foot) out at about 45 degrees from the center of your body. Slightly bend your knee, shifting your weight onto this foot. Reach both arms up to the left, stretching out your rib cage. Extend your right leg out to your right side with your toes pointed. Do not put any weight on this foot. Draw your elbows and right knee in toward the middle of your body at the same time, driving your arms and chest down to the right as your knee draws up diagonally between them. Crunch with your core. Extend your arms and leg back out and repeat for the proper interval time, then switch and perform the exercise with your left leg, extending out to your left side.

Too Hard?	*Too Easy?*
Don't raise your knee as high. Move slower.	Really bring that knee up and crunch harder. Move faster. Hold a dumbbell at its ends.

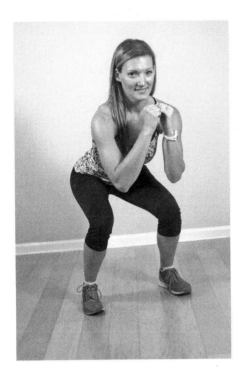
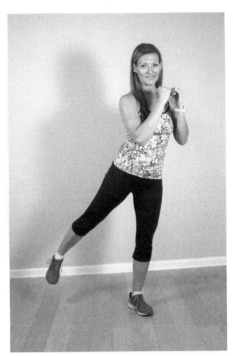

ALTERNATING SQUAT LIFTS

Stand with your feet hip width apart. Lower into a squat (¾ to parallel). As you rise up out of the squat, lift your right foot to the rear about 45 degrees, squeezing your glutes. Come back into the squat position. Rise up again and lift your left foot to the rear with the same glute squeeze. Keep alternating your legs throughout the interval time.

Too Hard?

Keep your squats shallow.

Too Easy?

Hold dumbbells on your shoulders.

Move faster.

Pulse squat at the bottom.

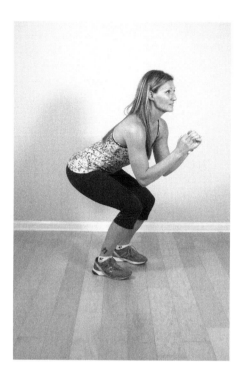 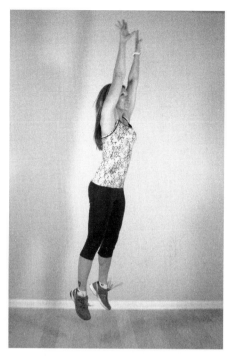

JUMP SQUATS

Stand with your feet hip width apart and your hands resting lightly on the tops of your thighs. Lower yourself into a deep squat no lower than parallel to the floor and jump up into the air. As you jump, lift your arms overhead as if you're trying to reach the ceiling or shoot a basketball. Land back into a deep squat and immediately repeat.

Too Hard?	*Too Easy?*
Do a normal squat.	Go lower into the squat.
	Jump higher.
	Take off from the floor faster.

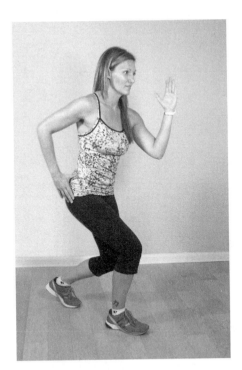
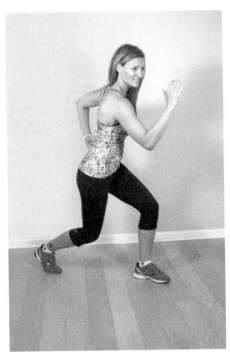

JAB STEPS (MOVING QUICKLY)

Start in a staggered stance with your right leg forward, your left leg back, and your knees bent. Hold your arms at your sides at 90-degree angles, as if you're about to take off running. Quickly step forward with your left foot. You should land in a slightly lunged position. Your right foot should remain stationary throughout the exercise on this side, but rise up on the ball of the foot as your left foot is landing. Now quickly retract your left foot, springing backward to the start position (still holding a slight lunge). Pump your arms back and forth with each step (as if you are sprinting). They will work in an opposite swing of your feet.

Too Hard?	*Too Easy?*
Slow down a little bit.	You're amazing! Hold a dumbbell in each hand.

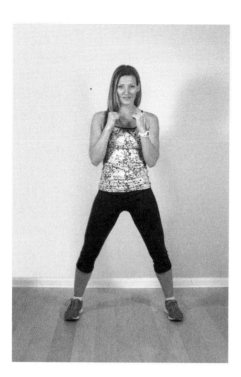
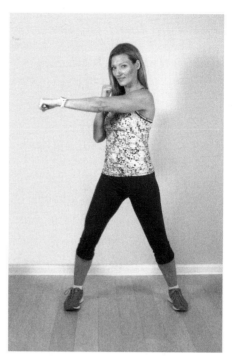

ALTERNATING TWIST WITH PUNCHES

Stand with your feet shoulder width apart with your knees slightly bent, making sure you keep your weight evenly distributed on both legs. Bring your fists near your chin and quickly turn your upper body to the right while you throw a punch with your left arm. Be sure to keep your hips straight, twisting only your upper body. Then turn to the left and punch with your right hand. Keep repeating, moving quickly from right to left. Keep your abs tight throughout the exercise.

Too Hard?

Slow down a little bit.

Too Easy?

Contract your abs harder.

Move faster.

Hold light dumbbells in each hand.

The Daily Lube

WHAT YOU NEED

An open space

A resistance band or tube (if you don't have either, a jump rope will work)

A yoga-style mat

Sneakers (optional)

What you need to know: This routine is meant to relax and stretch your muscles while maximizing your joint mobility. Each of these movements should be performed with loose muscles and fluidity. You should move seamlessly and slowly through each exercise from start to finish before moving on to the next one. You will do all of the exercises in sequence with your right leg before moving on to your left.

Take your time and relax. Don't bounce or push yourself to stretch beyond your capabilities. You will know if you are pushing a stretch too far because your leg will start to twitch. That's bad! Ease off the stretch and keep going at a more moderate level. And don't hold your breath! Your body requires oxygen at all times, and stretching isn't an exception. Breathing will help you relax and go deeper into the stretches. So stay ultra-relaxed and breathe normally throughout the entire routine.

Right now you're thinking, "Wait a sec! I thought there were only three workouts in this plan!" Well, you're right. The Daily Lube isn't a workout; it's a magic pill for muscle soreness and a thank-you to your body for all of its hard work.

Check out videos of all these exercises on my Web site, www.amycotta.com!

Pain, Pain, Go Away!

Imagine that your body is the Tin Man from *The Wizard of Oz,* and The Daily Lube is the oil that keeps you moving. This routine will loosen up the muscles deep within your hips, thighs, and glutes. The gentle dynamic movements will help combat soreness and keep you limber. A day or so after you begin the exercise program, you're going to need them!

A Word to the Wise

You can do these exercises as part of your normal daily routine, or you can perform them on your off days. The choice is yours. Just know that if you are doing the Blast, Firm, and Burn workouts correctly, you're going to want The Daily Lube, need The Daily Lube, and love The Daily Lube. If you find that's not the case, you're not working hard enough. To check out videos of all these exercises, visit my Web site www.amycotta.com!

LEG LIFTS

Lie flat on your back with your legs out straight. Place the resistance band on the arch of your right foot and choke up on it to add some tension. If the band is wiggly, it's too loose. Maintaining a constant fluid motion, lift your right leg vertically toward your chest, slightly pausing at the top position (wherever your body comfortably allows), before lowering your foot again. Perform all reps with this leg before moving on to the next exercise.

STATIC HOLD

Lying in the same position as the leg-lifts exercise, use the resistance device to pull your right leg up and as close to your body as you can to get a stretch. If your leg starts to shake, or if your knee starts to bend, back off the stretch until neither happens. Hold for 15 to 20 seconds before moving on to the next exercise.

OPEN LEG HOLD AND CIRCLES

Lie flat on your back with your legs out straight, imagining that your body is a clock, with your head at 12 and your feet at 6. With the resistance device across the bottom of your right foot, move your right leg out to the side at 4 and let it hang. Choke up on the band as needed to keep tension in the tubing. Hold for a count of 10 to 15 seconds. Then, holding this position, perform 8 to 15 circles in a clockwise direction, and 8 to 15 circles in a counterclockwise direction. Bring your leg back to the center of the body and move on to the next exercise.

IT-BAND STRETCH WITH CIRCLES

Lie on your back with your legs out straight. Keep both hips firmly on the ground. Move your right foot across your body to your left side (9 position). You will pass the midline of your body. You may not be able to take your leg over very far, and that's okay. Cross over only as far as you can without your hip coming off the floor. Hold for a count of 10 to 15 seconds. Then perform 8 to 15 small circles in a clockwise direction, and 8 to 15 circles in a counterclockwise direction. Once you have completed the circles, bring your leg up straight and release before moving on to the next exercise.

OPEN AND CLOSE THE DOOR

Lying flat on your back with your legs out straight, allow your right leg to drop back to your right side (4 position). Open up your hip as much as you can comfortably handle. Keeping your shoulders on the ground and your legs straight, move your leg all the way to your left side. At this point, you will be twisted like a pretzel. Your right hip will come off the ground (shoulders stay on the ground). Hold for a count of 15 to 20 seconds. Now slowly raise your leg straight up to the center of your body, with your foot pointed toward the ceiling, and allow it to swing back to the starting 4 position (to your right). Using a fluid movement, keep moving your leg through this pretzel movement, crossing your body each time. Repeat 8 times before moving on to the next exercise.

SWEEPING HIP CIRCLES

Lying flat on your back with your legs out straight, keeping your hips loose, make 8 to 15 large sweeping circles clockwise and 8 to 15 large sweeping circles counterclockwise with your right leg. Dip your foot low at the bottom of the circle and swing it back up high as you come back around. Keep your leg ultra-relaxed throughout the movement.

Now repeat all of these exercises in sequence with your left leg.

Skinny Jeans
ROCK ST★R

Before: Size 14   After: Size 12

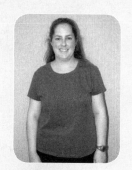

Name: Liza

Age: 38

Occupation: Payroll administrator

Children: None

Pounds lost: 10.5

What I learned: I'm much stronger than I thought I was. I also learned I can do anything, even a big challenge, if I set my mind to it.

What I want to share: I really enjoyed the ease of the program. It was tough to stick to the no-carb diet for the first week, but after the first week, I got used to the food choices and it became much easier. I was a little worried about adding in carbs at week 4, but I worked really hard to keep my carbs to a minimum. I can't say I enjoyed the workouts, because they honestly kicked my butt every time. However, I did enjoy the results from the workouts.

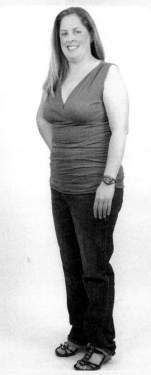

Chapter 6

THE DIET—IGNITE AND MELT

All right, sister! It's time to kick the tires and light the fire! I'm going to share with you the two-part eating plan that I've used for years when I needed to get myself in fitness-competition or camera-ready shape and lose weight after having babies. I'm no different from anyone else. I love to eat, and I love my beer. We all have cravings and weaknesses, but I assure you: If I can do it, you can, too!

The Skinny Jeans eating plan has been made as dummy-proof as possible. You'll find lists of which foods to eat and which foods to avoid in both the Ignite and Melt phases, meal plans with suggestions on what to chow down on throughout the day, and a collection of delicious recipes simple enough to make anytime. However, you are going to have to do a little work. As I mentioned in Chapter 1, you're going to keep a food log. You will find 42 blank food logs in Appendix I for every day of the program. Follow the directions starting on page 7 for keeping track of your food choices, calorie intake, and more.

(Okay, I can already hear you whining. But trust me: You've got this.)

IGNITE Your Fat Loss

Weeks 1, 2, 3

During the first 3 weeks, we are going to get you eating foods that will (alongside your daily workouts) help you say good-bye to flab! You will be taking in healthy, unsaturated fats; slow-burn carbohydrates; and high-quality proteins to aid in slowing down your digestion and help you achieve an overall lower glycemic index (GI). Insulin will slowly be released into your bloodstream, and your energy levels will remain stable so that you feel fuller longer between meals. As a result, you're going to lose weight and inches without feeling deprived or tired. The foods you'll be eating will be filling but not calorie dense, so you'll need to eat a larger quantity in order to hit your caloric goal. Make sure you are eating enough food. Believe it or not, eating too little is just as bad for your metabolism as overeating!

Think of your body as a car. Your car requires fuel in order to run. Food is your body's form of gasoline. Without gas in your tank (body), your motor (metabolism) will get sluggish and eventually slow down and stop. On the flip side, you don't want to take in more fuel (food) than your body requires, or you'll gain weight! The best way to lose weight is to feed your body throughout the day so that it burns off the calories as fuel without having any left over to be stored as fat.

As you'll see on the Skinny plate below, the major portion of your calories will be coming from high-quality slow-burn vegetables, followed by lean protein and dairy. With *Six Weeks to Skinny Jeans,* your main goal is to get your plate looking like the one on this page while hitting your daily caloric-intake goal. As discussed in The Diet Q&A (starting on page 3), you'll be filling any nutritional gaps with a multivitamin/mineral supplement.

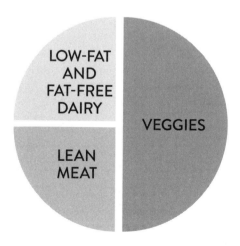

Excited yet? Following is a list of specific foods to enjoy and to avoid in the Ignite phase, based on their nutritional makeup.

CHEESE (Calcium for those awesome bones!)

Enjoy: Reduced-fat Cheddar or feta cheese, 1% or 2% cottage cheese, low-fat cream cheese, part-skim mozzarella, Parmesan cheese, low-fat ricotta, Laughing Cow Light cheese

Avoid: Any full-fat cheese or cream cheese

DRINKS (Hydration is key!)

Enjoy: Coffee (black or with fat-free milk), tea (green, black, or herbal), V8 tomato juice, regular or sparkling water

Avoid: Alcohol (beer, wine, liquor), sugary coffee drinks, energy drinks, fruit juice, soda

EGGS AND OTHER DAIRY PRODUCTS (Lean protein and/or calcium)

Enjoy: Eggs, liquid egg whites, fat-free milk, fat-free sour cream, I Can't Believe It's Not Butter! or Smart Balance Buttery Spread Made with Extra Virgin Olive Oil, fat-free plain or Greek yogurt, sugar-free yogurt

Avoid: Ice cream, all milk except fat-free, queso dip, full-fat sour cream. Also watch out for soy milk—most varieties have high sugar content

FRUIT (Vitamin C, baby!)

Enjoy: Lemons and limes

Avoid: All other fruits and fruit juices

HERBS AND SPICES

Enjoy: Basil, bay leaves, black pepper, cilantro, cumin, garlic, lemon pepper, oregano, paprika, parsley, sage, thyme

MEAT (Lean protein, iron)

Enjoy: Canadian bacon, low-sodium beef broth, lean beef tenderloin, bison, lean ground sirloin, lean sirloin steaks

Avoid: Regular bacon, fatty cuts of beef, ham with honey or maple, hamburger, jerky, veal

OILS, VINEGARS, AND CONDIMENTS

Enjoy: Balsamic vinegar, Dijon mustard, dill pickles, guacamole, hot sauce, extra-virgin olive oil, red wine vinegar, light salad dressing, Kraft Mayo with Olive Oil, sauerkraut, sesame oil, low-sodium soy sauce, low-sodium steak sauce, Tabasco sauce, tahini, tomato sauce (low sugar), Worcestershire sauce

Avoid: Regular butter, ketchup, lard, pasta sauce

POULTRY (Lean protein)

Enjoy: Low-sodium chicken broth, all white-meat turkey or chicken breast, deli turkey or chicken, turkey bacon, ground turkey or chicken breast

Avoid: Chicken wings or legs, duck or goose breast, processed poultry (nuggets or fingers)

SEAFOOD (Protein and healthy, omega-3 fats)

Enjoy: Canned crabmeat, halibut, mahimahi, salmon, scallops, shrimp, sole, swordfish, tilapia, tuna steak, water-packed canned tuna

SNACKS (Have a treat!)

Enjoy: Sugar-free ice pops, sugar-free pudding, and sugar-free gelatin desserts

Avoid: All cakes, cookies, doughnuts, pies—you know . . . all junk food! Also be careful with sugar-free candies; they have chemicals that can cause major gastrointestinal distress.

SOY, NUTS, BEANS (Protein, healthy fats, and fiber)

Enjoy: Almonds (dry roasted), black beans, chickpeas, edamame, hummus, pine nuts, pinto beans, pistachios, red kidney beans, seitan, tempeh, tofu, walnuts, white beans

Avoid: Cashews, macadamia nuts

STARCHES, CARBS, AND JUNK FOOD

Avoid: Baked goods (cookies, cakes, muffins, pies), all bread and bread products, candy, dry cereal, chips, fried food, oatmeal, pasta, all rice and rice products

VEGETABLES (**Vitamins, minerals, and fiber**)

Enjoy: Artichokes, asparagus, avocado, bell peppers, broccoli, cabbage, cauliflower, celery, cucumbers, collard greens, eggplant, green beans, green

GI FOODS LIST: FOR YOUR SIX WEEKS TO SKINNY JEANS JOURNEY AND BEYOND

LOW—less than 40

Fruits: cherries, grapefruit, peaches, plums

Grains: pearled barley, rice bran

Sugars: fructose

Vegetables: peas (dried), soybeans

Other: milk chocolate, peanuts, yogurt (sugar-free, plain)

MODERATE—40 to 60

Grains: corn hominy, oats, whole grain pancakes, whole wheat pasta, brown rice, rye

Vegetables: black-eyed peas, raw carrots, green beans, lima beans, starchy beans (white, black, brown, kidney, pinto, chickpeas), tomato soup

Fruits: apples, apricots, oranges, dried pears

Other: ice cream, fettuccine, milk (all), spaghetti, ravioli, vermicelli, yogurt (with sugar)

MODERATELY HIGH—60 to 80

Grains: buckwheat, bran, pumpernickel

Vegetables: baked beans, green peas, sweet potatoes, yams

bell peppers, lemons, lettuce (all types), mixed greens, mushrooms, onions, spinach, snow peas, squash, tomatoes, zucchini

Avoid: Beets, carrots, corn, white or sweet potatoes, yams

ABSOLUTELY FORBIDDEN

If it's dipped, fried, or otherwise filled with sugar or fat, avoid it like the plague.

Fruits: grapes, kiwifruit, pears, pineapple

Other: devil's food or sponge cake, fruit juice, oatmeal raisin cookies, potato chips

HIGH—80 to 100

Grains: rye bread, wheat bread, white bread, corn tortilla, sweet corn, cream of wheat, Grape-Nuts, white rice

Vegetables: mashed or boiled white potatoes, new potatoes

Sugars: sucrose

Fruits: apricots, bananas, mangoes, papaya, raisins

Other: cookies, corn chips, crackers, energy bars, pastries, cheese pizza

EXTREMELY HIGH—100+

Grains: french bread, cornflakes, millet, instant potatoes, instant rice, puffed rice

Vegetables: cooked carrots, fava beans, parsnips, baked white potatoes

Sugars: glucose, honey, maltrose

Fruits: watermelon

Other: Cheerios, doughnuts, french fries, pretzels, rice cakes, waffles

Using the MELT Plan

Weeks 4, 5, 6

At this point, you will be seeing some *major* improvements in your body and in the way your clothes fit. But, oh sister, we are not done yet. Since we've Ignited your fat loss, we're now going to Melt away the remaining fluff from that hot little body of yours. The Melt plan is designed to last for the remaining 3 weeks as you continue to lose inches. You'll eat the same foods as in the Ignite plan, but you're able to add in some medium- and faster-burning carbs.

A friendly warning: This portion of the diet is *not*—I repeat, *not*—a Carba-palooza. You're not going to eat every piece of fruit or whole wheat bread in sight. If you do, we might as well go back to week 1.

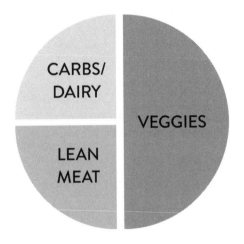

The Melt Breakdown

You may still enjoy everything allowed on the Ignite meal plan while adding in these foods.

FRUIT (In moderation)

Enjoy: Apples, blueberries, blackberries, cantaloupe, cherries, grapefruits, grapes, kiwifruit, oranges, peaches, pears, plums, prunes, raspberries, strawberries

Avoid: Bananas, dates, figs, canned fruit, fruit juices, mangoes, papaya, pineapple, raisins, watermelon

GRAINS AND STARCHY CARBS (In moderation; stay within your plate proportion and caloric goal)

Enjoy: Light whole wheat and multigrain bread products, raw carrots,* Fiber One cereal, egg fettuccine, slow-cooked oats, whole wheat pasta, sweet potatoes, brown rice, yams

Avoid: White-flour products, including but not limited to white bread, biscuits, hamburger buns, cooked carrots,* corn meal, couscous, crackers, croissants, pancakes, pasta, white potatoes, pretzels, rice cakes, white rice, dinner rolls, taco shells, tapioca

In the Melt phase, you can eat low- and moderate-GI foods (see "GI Food List," pages 120–121).

---

*You may have raw carrots in the Melt phase; however, because the cooking process spikes their GI, cooked carrots are off-limits.

Skinny Jeans
ROCK ST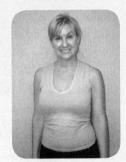R

Before: Size 4–6   After: Size 2

Name: Stephanie

Age: 41

Occupation: Entertainment and model agent

Children: 1

Pounds lost: 6

What I was afraid of: I was afraid I wouldn't have the discipline to follow the plan.

What I liked: Six Weeks to Skinny Jeans taught me to love exercise again.

What I learned: I am a carb addict! I also learned how to lose that addiction and like more foods than those with just flour and sugar. I can eat a lot less calories and love the food I eat!

What I want to share: I am exercising more than I have in the last 8 years and am working on changing my eating habits for life!

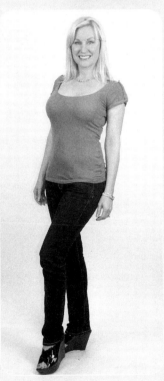

Chapter 7

SKINNY RECIPES

A girl's got to eat!

That means a girl has to cook. These recipes taste great and are quick and easy to prepare, which means getting back into your Skinny Jeans has never been easier!

All the Six Weeks to Skinny Jeans recipes have been tried and tested on America's pickiest eaters, my family. They all passed with flying colors and I know you and your family will enjoy them as well. So flip through the recipes, dust off the sauté pan, and get cooking!

For more recipes and cooking tips, visit my Web site www.amycotta.com.

SOUPS

Skinny Vegetable Soup

IGNITE
and
MELT

This light, savory soup is packed with fiber for a delicious, system-cleansing meal addition or snack. It can be prepared with any of the vegetables allowed in the Ignite phase. Make the entire recipe and freeze individual servings to have on hand.

Makes 18 servings

¼ medium white onion, chopped

2 teaspoons minced garlic

1 cup each (5 maximum) of the following fresh vegetables, chopped: bean sprouts, bell peppers, broccoli, cabbage, cauliflower, celery, eggplant, green beans, mushrooms, spinach, squash, zucchini

3 cups skinned and diced fresh tomatoes

2 quarts low-sodium chicken broth (homemade or with no MSG or preservatives)

1 quart water

Salt and pepper

Soy sauce (optional)

Heat a large skillet over medium-high heat and coat with cooking spray. Add the onion and garlic and cook for 2 to 3 minutes, stirring often, until tender. Add the vegetables of your choice, one by one, from hardest to softest, and cook each for 1 minute before adding the next one. Add the tomatoes last, and cook for 1 minute.

Transfer the vegetables to a large soup pot and add the chicken broth and water. Cover and simmer for about 20 minutes, seasoning with salt and pepper to taste. Add a little bit of soy sauce if you would like before serving.

Note: *Also check the broth label for "variants" of MSG, like hydrolyzed soy protein, whey protein, autolyzed yeast, and yeast extract.*

Per serving: 20 calories, 1 gram protein, 4 grams carbohydrates, 0 gram fat, 1 gram fiber, 57 milligrams sodium

Skinny Scallop Soup

This light, flavorful seafood soup is easy to make and can be served as a meal by itself or with the Skinny Colorful Salad for added fiber. You can substitute frozen (thawed) asparagus for fresh spears.

IGNITE *and* **MELT**

Makes 4 servings

- 5 cups low-sodium chicken broth
- 3 tablespoons chopped fresh cilantro
- 2 teaspoons lemon zest
- ¼ teaspoon black pepper
- 12 ounces fresh or frozen bay scallops, thawed and rinsed

- 1 pound fresh asparagus spears, trimmed and chopped into bite-size pieces
- 1 cup sliced fresh mushrooms
- ½ cup chopped green onion
- 1 tablespoon lemon juice

In a large saucepan, combine the broth, cilantro, lemon zest, and pepper. Bring to a boil and add the scallops, asparagus, mushrooms, and green onion. Reduce the heat to medium-high and simmer, uncovered, for 3 to 5 minutes, until the asparagus is tender and the scallops are opaque. Remove from the heat and add the lemon juice.

Per serving: 129 calories, 20 grams protein, 11 grams carbohydrates, 1 gram fat, 3 grams fiber, 231 milligrams sodium

SALADS

Skinny Colorful Salad

IGNITE
and
MELT

This quick salad is full of color and crunch. The chickpeas are a great, protein-packed alternative to meat, which makes it a perfect choice for vegetarians. Enjoy alone or with any of the Skinny soups for a full meal.

Makes 8 servings

Dressing

- ¼ cup extra-virgin olive oil
- 2 tablespoons red wine vinegar
- 1 teaspoon kosher salt
- 2 packages sugar substitute (Splenda, stevia, or Truvia)
- 1 teaspoon minced garlic

Salad

- 5 medium plum tomatoes, chopped
- 1 can (15 ounces) chickpeas, drained
- 1 medium cucumber, peeled and cubed
- 1 large green bell pepper, chopped
- 1 cup chopped fresh cilantro
- ¼ cup finely chopped chives

To make the dressing: In a small jar or lidded container, combine the olive oil, vinegar, salt, sugar substitute, and garlic. Shake to blend. Set aside.

To make the salad: In a large bowl, combine the tomatoes, chickpeas, cucumber, bell pepper, cilantro, and chives. Drizzle with the dressing and toss.

Per serving: 111 calories, 2½ grams protein, 9 grams carbohydrates, 8 grams fat, 2 grams fiber, 323 milligrams sodium

Skinny Palm Salad

This tropical low-calorie salad is great for the girl on the go. Toss it into a plastic to-go container and you're out the door. Hearts of palm should be available in the jarred-food aisle of most grocery stores. Top with some grilled chicken or salmon for added protein, or, if you're in the Melt phase, jazz it up with some baby spinach and sliced strawberries.

IGNITE *and* **MELT**

Makes 4 servings

6 cups mixed salad greens, rinsed

1 can (14 ounces) hearts of palm, drained and chopped

¼ cup reduced-fat olive oil–vinaigrette dressing or ½ teaspoon extra-virgin olive oil and ½ teaspoon balsamic vinegar

In a large salad bowl, combine the greens and hearts of palm. Drizzle with the dressing or the olive oil and vinegar and toss.

Per serving: 57 calories, 3 grams protein, 7 grams carbohydrates, 3 grams fat, 3 grams fiber, 403 milligrams sodium

ENTRÉES

Skinny Mexican Stir-Fry

This dish is a real crowd-pleaser: No one will know that this is a diet food! Turn up the heat with jalapeño chile peppers or add a little crunch by wrapping each serving in a large lettuce leaf. If you're in the Melt phase, you can add brown rice for extra flavor and texture.

Makes 4 servings

2 tablespoons extra-virgin olive oil

16 ounces lean turkey breast, cut into bite-size chunks

3 garlic cloves, minced

1 cup chopped onion

1 can (7 ounces) chopped green chiles, drained

1 medium red bell pepper, chopped

1 jalapeño pepper, seeded and chopped (optional)

½ cup no salt added tomato sauce

1 teaspoon chili powder

2 tablespoons chopped fresh cilantro (optional)

Heat 1 tablespoon of the oil in a large nonstick skillet. Add the turkey and sauté for about 7 minutes, or until it is fully cooked. Remove the turkey and set to the side. Add the remaining 1 tablespoon oil and the garlic, onion, chiles, bell pepper, jalapeño pepper (if using), tomato sauce, and chili powder. Cook, stirring, for about 5 minutes, or until the onions are soft.

Add the cilantro and turkey. Simmer for 2 to 3 minutes longer. Serve over greens or, if you are in the Melt phase, ½ cup brown rice.

Per serving (without rice): 228 calories, 29 grams protein, 10 grams carbohydrates, 9 grams fat, 2 grams fiber, 216 milligrams sodium

Skinny Frittata

When plain eggs just won't do, try this flavorful crustless quiche! This is a Melt splurge because of the quinoa or whole wheat flour and the full-fat cheese. I like Bob's Red Mill quinoa flour, which is available at Walmart and Whole Foods. You may also substitute low-fat feta cheese for the goat cheese. Enjoy!

MELT ONLY

Makes 8 servings

2 whole eggs

6 egg whites

½ cup fat-free milk

½ cup quinoa or whole wheat flour

1 teaspoon baking powder

2 cups 2% cottage cheese

1½ cups crumbled goat cheese (or low-fat feta cheese)

1 teaspoon salt

1 cup seeded, finely chopped green pepper

4 medium zucchini, sliced into thin half-moons

3 cups sliced mushrooms

2 cups spinach

1 small onion, peeled and sliced

2 garlic cloves, minced

½ teaspoon chopped fresh basil

½ teaspoon black pepper

Preheat the oven to 400°F. In a large bowl, beat the eggs and egg whites and stir in the milk, flour, baking powder, cottage cheese, 1 cup of the goat cheese, and ½ teaspoon of the salt. Set aside.

In a large nonstick skillet, sauté the green pepper, zucchini, mushrooms, spinach, onion, and garlic and cook for 2 to 5 minutes, until the vegetables are tender. Add the cooked vegetables to the egg mixture and mix in the basil, pepper, and the remaining salt.

Coat a large casserole dish with olive oil cooking spray. Pour the mixture into the dish and top with the remaining goat cheese. Bake for 20 minutes, then lower the oven temperature to 350°F and bake for 45 minutes longer, or until a knife comes out clean from the center.

Note: *You can also make individual servings by pouring the mixture into the cups of a muffin pan instead of a casserole dish.*

Per serving: 216 calories, 19 grams protein, 17 grams carbohydrates, 9 grams fat, 3 grams fiber, 750 milligrams sodium

Skinny Minis

These bite-size egg muffins might be small, but they're mighty! Each is packed with 11 grams of high-quality protein! Enjoy them for breakfast or pack them up in your lunch. Want a little kick? Drizzle some hot sauce on them before serving. Yum!

Makes 8 servings

6 slices Canadian bacon

1 cup fat-free Cheddar cheese (shredded)

6 eggs

4 egg whites

2 tablespoons fat-free milk

¼ teaspoon pepper

Heat the oven to 375°F. Coat the muffin cups in a muffin pan with cooking spray. Cut the bacon into fourths and divide the pieces up evenly in the bottoms of the muffin cups. Divide the cheese evenly on top of the bacon in the muffin cups. Mix the eggs, egg whites, milk, and pepper. Pour the mixture evenly into the muffin cups. Bake for 20 to 25 minutes, until a knife comes out clean from the center of the egg muffin.

Per serving: 118 calories, 15 grams protein, 2 grams carbohydrates, 5 grams fat, 0 gram fiber, 479 milligrams sodium

Skinny Stuffed Red Peppers

This dish is a favorite at my house—even my pickiest eaters who won't eat peppers in any other setting love them in this recipe. The baking of the peppers brings out a sweetness that makes you forget that you're eating a healthy vegetable. If you want to make your serving platter look and taste even more inviting, use a combination of red, yellow, and green bell peppers. Add the Skinny Colorful Salad (see page 128), and you've got a tasty meal that is packed with nutrition.

IGNITE
and
MELT

Makes 4 servings

2 teaspoons olive oil

½ cup chopped onion

½ cup chopped celery

1 clove garlic

1¼ pounds ground turkey

1 egg or egg substitute

1 teaspoon Italian seasoning

¼ teaspoon garlic powder

Salt and pepper

4 large red bell peppers, deseeded and sliced in half lengthwise

1 can (8 ounces) no salt added tomato sauce

1 can (14½ ounces) Italian diced tomatoes

¼ cup grated reduced-fat mozzarella cheese

Set the oven at 350°F. Heat the olive oil in a nonstick pan over medium heat. Add the onion, celery, and garlic and sauté for 5 to 10 minutes, until the vegetables are tender. Set aside.

In a mixing bowl, combine the turkey, egg or egg substitute, Italian seasoning, garlic powder, and salt and pepper to taste. Mix well. Fold the vegetables into the turkey mixture. Stuff the mixture into the pepper halves.

In another mixing bowl, combine the tomato sauce and diced tomatoes (with liquid). Pour the mixture over the pepper halves, making sure they are covered well. Sprinkle the tops of the peppers with ⅛ cup of the cheese. Cover with foil and bake for 50 minutes.

Uncover the peppers, sprinkle on the remaining ⅛ cup of the cheese and bake for 10 minutes longer before serving.

Per serving: 296 calories, 42 grams protein, 22 grams carbohydrates, 5 grams fat, 6 grams fiber, 471 milligrams sodium

Skinny Beef Kebobs

IGNITE
and
MELT

Kebobs are a fun alternative to your typical steak or chicken breast. Feel free to substitute chicken, shrimp, or scallops for the beef. If you are looking for a great vegetarian dish, look no further! Nix the meat and use tofu; portobello mushrooms; and sliced zucchini, squash, and onions.

Makes 6 servings

Marinade

3 green onions, sliced

¼ cup extra-virgin olive oil

3 tablespoons lemon juice

1½ teaspoons minced garlic

2 teaspoons dried tarragon

½ teaspoon dried oregano

¼ teaspoon black pepper

Kebobs

1½ pounds beef sirloin steak, cubed and trimmed of fat

To make the marinade: In a small bowl, combine the onions, oil, lemon juice, garlic, tarragon, oregano, and pepper. Pour into a large resealable plastic bag, add the meat, and seal. Place the bag in a shallow bowl and refrigerate for 4 to 24 hours. Drain and discard remaining marinade.

To make the kebobs: Preheat the oven to broil. Put the meat cubes onto metal kebob skewers, leaving about ¼ inch between cubes. Place the kebobs on a cool broiler pan and cook for 10 to 12 minutes, until the inside of the meat is browned or just slightly pink.

Per serving: 336 calories, 23 grams protein, 2 grams carbohydrates, 26 grams fat, 0 gram fiber, 59 milligrams sodium

Skinny Stroganoff

Want to feel like a rebel on your diet? Try some of this hearty concoction, and you'll think you've died and gone to bad-food heaven. This is a rich-tasting dish without all the calories and fat of traditional Stroganoff. The egg noodles make it a Melt option only.

MELT ONLY

Makes 2 servings

1 cup whole wheat egg noodles

½ pound lean ground sirloin, cubed

1 can (10¾ ounces) fat-free cream of mushroom soup

1 tablespoon reduced-fat sour cream

½ cup sliced mushrooms

Boil water and cook the pasta as directed on the package. Drain and transfer back to the pot.

Heat a large nonstick skillet over medium-high heat and cook the beef, stirring constantly, until thoroughly browned. Drain excess fat from the pan and mix in the mushroom soup, sour cream, and mushrooms. Turn the burner to low heat and simmer for about 5 minutes.

Stir the meat mixture into the pasta and serve.

Per serving: 360 calories, 31 grams protein, 32 grams carbohydrates, 13 grams fat, 5 grams fiber, 137 milligrams sodium

Skinny Waffles

MELT
ONLY

Waffles and smiles, oh my! Indulge in this awesome breakfast treat. The whole wheat flour makes these waffles wholesome and fiber-licious, and they get their sweetness from the applesauce and sugar substitute. They're delicious without syrup, but you may use a drizzle of sugar-free or low-sugar syrup to take them to the next level in taste. If you're feeling daring, top with your favorite sliced berries. You will need to account for the extra calories if using syrup or topping with fruit.

Makes 5 servings

1¾ cups whole wheat flour

½ teaspoon salt

1 tablespoon baking powder

3 teaspoons sugar substitute
(Splenda, stevia, or Truvia)

2 egg yolks

1¾ cups fat-free milk

½ cup unsweetened applesauce

1 teaspoon vanilla extract

2 egg whites

Preheat the waffle maker. In a large mixing bowl, combine the flour, salt, baking powder and sugar substitute.

In a smaller bowl, combine the egg yolks, milk, applesauce, and vanilla. Place the egg whites into their own small mixing bowl and set aside.

Combine the liquid ingredients with the dry ingredients in the large bowl and mix well. Beat the egg whites until they peak. Gently fold the egg whites into the bowl with the other ingredients (don't overmix).

Coat the waffle maker with cooking spray. Pour the batter into the waffle maker and cook for 3 to 5 minutes, until the waffle is lightly browned. Repeat with the remaining batter.

Per serving (without syrup or topping): 219 calories, 11 grams protein, 40 grams carbohydrates, 3 grams fat, 5 grams fiber, 559 milligrams sodium

Skinny Lettuce Wraps

Craving fish tacos? Try this light, crispy substitute. You may swap the tuna for ground turkey, extra-lean ground beef, shrimp, grilled fish, portobello mushrooms, or tofu. If you are in the Melt phase, try wrapping with a whole wheat tortilla instead of a lettuce leaf. Just make sure you account for the calorie difference (you can check calories at www.myfitnesspal.com).

IGNITE
and
MELT

Makes 1 serving

1 can (6 ounces) water-packed low-sodium tuna, drained and rinsed

½ cup no salt added pinto beans, drained and rinsed

⅛ avocado, sliced

½ cup fresh, diced tomato

Lemon juice (optional)

4 large romaine lettuce leaves, rinsed

Break up the tuna in a mixing bowl. Microwave the beans for 1 minute and combine with the tuna. Mix in the avocado, tomato, and lemon juice to taste (if using). Spoon the mixture evenly inside the lettuce leaves. Roll the leaves and serve like wraps.

Per serving: 358 calories, 50 grams protein, 27 grams carbohydrates, 6 grams fat, 11 grams fiber, 127 milligrams sodium

SNACKS AND SIDES

Skinny Parmesan Artichoke Hearts

IGNITE
and
MELT

This is a quick, low-calorie side dish totally bursting with flavor. Serve with chicken, steak, or fish or throw on top of a salad for a tangy, cheesy zing.

Makes 3 hearts per 1 serving

1 jar (32 ounces) artichoke hearts (halves)

Salt and pepper

¼ cup grated Parmesan cheese

Heat the oven to 375°F. Cover a cookie sheet with foil. Drain and rinse the artichokes. If they are not already in halves, cut them into halves.

Coat the foil with cooking spray. Place the artichokes evenly across the cookie sheet and coat the artichokes lightly with cooking spray. Sprinkle ⅛ cup of the cheese on top of the artichokes, setting aside the other ⅛ cup. Add the salt and pepper to taste.

Bake for 10 minutes, or until the artichokes are lightly golden brown. Remove from the oven, sprinkle the remaining ⅛ cup cheese on the artichokes, and serve.

Per serving: 52 calories, 4 grams protein, 6 grams carbohydrates, 2 grams fat, 2 grams fiber, 442 milligrams sodium

Skinny Crab-Deviled Eggs

These eggs make great little finger foods that you can pack and carry with you in your lunch box or take to your next luncheon or party. For optimal nutrition and taste, I like to use Kraft Mayo with Olive Oil instead of traditional mayonnaise. No one will ever know it's your diet food. Not a crab lover? You can swap out the entire ingredients list for hummus. Hollow out the hard-boiled eggs and fill them with your favorite flavored hummus. The calories will vary depending on the caloric content of the hummus you use.

IGNITE *and* **MELT**

Makes 8 servings

4 large hard-boiled eggs

4 teaspoons mayonnaise

1 teaspoon Dijon mustard

1 tablespoon chopped green onions

¼ cup lump crabmeat, shells removed

Cut the eggs lengthwise. Remove the yolks and place them in a mixing bowl. Mash with a fork and stir in the mayonnaise and mustard. Fold in the green onion. Spoon about a tablespoon of the mixture into each egg white half and top with the crabmeat.

Per serving: 52 calories, 4 grams protein, 1 gram carbohydrates, 4 grams fat, 0 gram fiber, 80 milligrams sodium

Skinny Squash

IGNITE
and
MELT

This is an awesome low-calorie, low-fat side dish for chicken, steak, fish, or pork. It's so hearty and delicious, you can even fill up your plate and make it a meal.

Makes 4 servings

1 medium tomato

2 small or 1 large zucchini, sliced thin

2 small or 1 large summer squash, sliced thin

2 tablespoons chopped green onion

1 teaspoon lemon juice

2 tablespoons extra-virgin olive oil

¾ teaspoon garlic powder

¼ teaspoon dried oregano

⅛ teaspoon pepper

2 tablespoons Parmesan cheese (grated)

Salt

Heat the oven to 350°F. Place the tomato, zucchini, squash, and onion in a small casserole dish. In a small bowl, combine the lemon juice, oil, garlic powder, oregano, and pepper.

Pour the mixture over the vegetables and toss so that they are properly coated. Heat for 20 to 30 minutes, until vegetables are al dente (lightly crisp). Sprinkle with the cheese and salt to taste and serve.

Per serving: 104 calories, 3 grams protein, 6 grams carbohydrates, 8 grams fat, 2 grams fiber, 47 milligrams sodium

Skinny Cucumber Salsa

This salsa is a fabulous vegetable dipper or complement to grilled chicken or fish. The cucumbers add a fresh summer crunch, while the lime and cilantro bring the zing. Want to sweeten it up? Spoon in a bit of agave syrup. Want to burn down the house? Add some extra jalapeño chile pepper.

IGNITE
and
MELT

Makes 6 servings

3 medium to large cucumbers, deseeded and diced

3 small to medium tomatoes, diced

1 medium green bell pepper, diced

2 jalapeño chile peppers, minced

½ cup chopped red onion

2 tablespoons minced cilantro

2 tablespoons minced fresh dill (optional)

3 squeezes of lime juice (fresh or bottled)

Combine the cucumbers, tomatoes, bell pepper, jalapeño chile peppers, and onion in a small mixing bowl. Add the cilantro; dill, if using; and lime juice and mix well. Chill before serving.

Per serving: 35 calories, 2 grams protein, 8 grams carbohydrates, 0 gram fat, 3 grams fiber, 4 milligrams sodium

Skinny Garlic Broccoli

IGNITE
and
MELT

This is a great side dish to accompany any dinner. The red pepper and oregano give it such a zesty flavor, you'll want to fill your plate! Add sliced almonds for a little crunch and healthy fat.

Makes 4 servings

2 teaspoons extra-virgin olive oil

2 cups (1 pound) broccoli florets, steamed and chopped

3 cloves of garlic, minced

¼ teaspoon dried oregano

¼ cup roasted red pepper, julienned

Heat the olive oil in a large nonstick skillet over medium-high heat. Add the broccoli, garlic, and oregano and sauté for about 3 minutes, or until the garlic is golden brown. Add the peppers and stir frequently for about 2 minutes, or until they are heated.

Per serving: 58 calories, 3 grams protein, 9 grams carbohydrates, 2 grams fat, 2 grams fiber, 113 milligrams sodium

Skinny Guacamole

This dip brings all the taste of restaurant guacamole at a fraction of the calories. Serve with sliced cucumbers, bell peppers and zucchini to dunk, or use it to add extra flavor and texture to the Skinny Mexican Stir-Fry (page 130) and Skinny Lettuce Wraps (page 137).

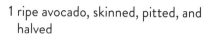

Makes 6 servings

1 ripe avocado, skinned, pitted, and halved

2 plum tomatoes, chopped

2 white or light green scallions, thinly sliced

1 small jalapeño chile pepper, seeded and minced

1 tablespoon lime juice

¼ teaspoon salt

In a small mixing bowl, mash the avocado with a fork. Add the tomatoes, scallions, pepper, lime juice, and salt. Mix well. Chill before serving.

Per serving: 45 calories, 1 gram protein, 3 grams carbohydrates, 4 grams fat, 2 grams fiber, 101 milligrams sodium

Skinny Zucchini Fries

If you've been dying for french fries, these crunchy munchies will kick your craving! They make a great side dish for any meal. Want to have a healthy BBQ? Pair up the fries with an extra-lean ground sirloin or ground turkey burger wrapped in a large lettuce leaf. Yummy!

Makes 2 servings

¼ cup grated Parmesan cheese

¼ cup egg substitute or egg whites

1 medium zucchini, rinsed and thinly sliced

Preheat the oven to 425°F.

Pour the Parmesan cheese into a resealable plastic bag. Pour the egg substitute or egg whites into a small bowl. Using a fork, submerge the zucchini slices in the egg and let the excess drip off. Place the egg-covered slices into the bag, close the bag, and shake until the cheese coats the zucchini.

Lightly coat a large cooking sheet with cooking spray. Lay the zucchini slices on the sheet and cook for 15 minutes, or until the cheese is lightly browned.

Per serving: 92 calories, 10 grams protein, 4 grams carbohydrates, 5 grams fat, 1 gram fiber, 320 milligrams sodium

SAUCES AND DRESSINGS

Skinny Marinade (for Beef and Chicken)

This zesty combo of herbs and spices is simple to prepare and will kick up the flavor of your meat in no time. I like to use Dale's Steak Seasoning for this recipe, but you are welcome to use your personal favorite.

IGNITE
and
MELT

Makes 4 servings

2 tablespoons dried onion

2 tablespoons minced garlic

1 tablespoon steak seasoning

½ teaspoon hickory-smoked salt

3 tablespoons water (for chicken only)

For beef: In a small mixing bowl, combine the onion, garlic, steak seasoning, and salt. With a pastry brush, brush this mixture onto steaks or any other kind of beef. Let the meat rest, covered, for 15 minutes before grilling or cooking on a skillet.

For chicken: In a small mixing bowl, combine the onion, garlic, steak seasoning, and salt. Add the water and pour the mixture into a resealable plastic bag. Add the chicken pieces to the bag and close tightly. Let the chicken rest for 30 minutes before baking or grilling.

Per serving: 15 calories, 0 gram protein, 3 grams carbohydrates, 0 gram fat, 1 gram fiber, 745 milligrams sodium

Skinny Roasted-Tomato Sauce

IGNITE and MELT

Who said you can't have your low-GI diet and your tomato sauce, too? This sauce is rich and satisfying, without all the added sugar and sodium of most store-bought brands. Serve it with some oven-baked eggplant and low-fat Italian cheese for a great, healthy-tasting eggplant parmigiana. In the Melt phase, mix it with whole wheat pasta. Mmm, mmm good!

Makes 5 servings

1 large sweet onion, halved lengthwise and sliced crosswise

3 pounds plum tomatoes (about 18), cut lengthwise into fourths

2 teaspoons extra-virgin olive oil

1 tablespoon balsamic vinegar

3 garlic cloves, minced

¾ teaspoon salt

¼ teaspoon black pepper

Preheat the oven to 375°F. Spray 2 large cookie sheets with cooking spray and arrange the onion and tomatoes on top in a single layer. Drizzle with the olive oil and vinegar and sprinkle on the garlic, salt, and pepper.

Roast for 50 to 55 minutes, switching sheets on the shelves (from top to bottom) halfway through the cooking time. The onions should be lightly browned when done. Remove the tomatoes and onions from the sheets and pulse in a food processor until the mixture is of a slightly chunky, sauce consistency.

Per serving: 78 calories, 3 grams protein, 14 grams carbohydrates, 3 grams fat, 4 grams fiber, 353 milligrams sodium

Skinny Blue Cheese Dressing

Even though this recipe calls for full-fat cheese, it contains only a fraction of the fat and calories of regular bottled blue cheese dressing, and none of the additives. Enjoy this creamy concoction on salads or as dip for sliced veggies.

MELT
ONLY

Makes 6 servings

½ cup low-fat buttermilk

2 teaspoons reduced-fat
   mayonnaise

2 tablespoons crumbled blue cheese

¼ teaspoon minced garlic

   Ground red pepper

2 teaspoons minced chives

Using a food processor or blender, mix the buttermilk, mayonnaise, cheese, and garlic and the pepper to taste. Pulse until the mixture is a semismooth consistency. Add the chives and combine with a spoon. Refrigerate the mixture in a covered container for at least 30 minutes before serving.

Per serving: 36 calories, 1 gram protein, 2 grams carbohydrates, 3 grams fat, 0 gram fiber, 102 milligrams sodium

Skinny Ketchup

IGNITE and MELT

Make this key condiment yourself and avoid all the sugar and chemicals of regular ketchup. Drizzle on top of burgers, meat loaf, or eggs.

Makes 20 servings

1 small can (6 ounces) of tomato paste

¼ cup cider vinegar

½ cup water

¼ teaspoon sea salt

⅛ teaspoon ground cloves

⅛ teaspoon ground cinnamon

⅛ teaspoon garlic powder

5 packets sugar substitute (Splenda, stevia, or Truvia)

Combine the tomato paste, vinegar, water, salt, cloves, cinnamon, garlic powder, and sugar substitute in a small bowl and mix until fully blended. Cover and refrigerate for at least 20 minutes before serving.

Per serving: 9 calories, 0 grams protein, 2 grams carbohydrates, 0 gram fat, 0 gram fiber, 84 milligrams sodium

DESSERTS

Skinny Chocolate Delight

This low-calorie, protein-packed chocolate dessert will put you back in your happy place without putting you back in your fat jeans. Close your eyes while you're eating it, and you'll forget that you're on a diet!

IGNITE
and
MELT

Makes 2 servings

½ cup 2% cottage cheese (you can also use ricotta cheese for a thicker consistency)

2 tablespoons unsweetened cocoa powder

2 tablespoons agave nectar

1 teaspoon cinnamon

Whisk the cottage cheese, cocoa powder, agave nectar, and cinnamon together in a mixing bowl or combine in a blender or food processor. Cover and chill for at least 10 minutes before serving.

Per serving: 116 calories, 7 grams protein, 23 grams carbohydrates, 1½ grams fat, 3 grams fiber, 211 milligrams sodium

Skinny Ice Pop

Indulge in one of these icy treats, and you'll never know you're not eating the tasty, drippy ice pops you loved as a kid. These are a great treat on a hot day or when you're jonesing for something sweet. If you're in the Melt phase, add thin slices of strawberries to filled cups before freezing.

Makes 16 servings

1 package (0.23 ounce) Kool-Aid Invisible Watermelon Kiwi Unsweetened Soft Drink Mix

1 cup sugar substitute (granulated)

2 quarts water

16 plastic or paper cups (5 ounces)

16 ice pop sticks

Combine the drink mix, sugar substitute, and water in a large pitcher and stir until dissolved. Pour the mixture into plastic cups, filling them evenly until the drink mix is gone. Place the cups in the freezer for about 1½ hours, or until the mixture is firm. Remove, insert the sticks into the cups, and then return to freezer for 1½ hours longer before serving.

Per serving (without added fruit): 6 calories, 0 gram protein, 2 grams carbohydrates, 0 gram fat, 0 gram fiber, 5 milligrams sodium

Skinny Parfait

Who doesn't love a sweet, creamy, totally decadent parfait? Not only is this one yummy, but it's also packed with high-quality protein. If you are in the Melt phase, feel free to add your (approved) fruit of choice. This recipe makes a fair amount, so you might want to stick some in the fridge for later. But if you're really hungry—eat up!

IGNITE and MELT

Makes 1 serving

5 ounces plain 2% greek yogurt

1 teaspoon ground cinnamon

½ ounce sliced almonds

½ tablespoon agave nectar

Mix the yogurt, cinnamon, almonds, and agave nectar into a small bowl and serve.

Per serving: 199 calories, 17 grams protein, 18 grams carbohydrates, 7 grams fat, 3 grams fiber, 0 milligrams sodium

Skinny Brown Sugar Apples

MELT ONLY

This fruity delight will satisfy even your most powerful sweet tooth. Eat it alone or as a topping on your Skinny Waffles. For a little extra wow, try it with the Skinny Fruit Dip (page 154).

Makes 1 serving

1 medium apple (any type), cored and sliced

½ tablespoon Splenda Brown Sugar Blend

½ tablespoon water

Lightly coat a nonstick pan with cooking spray and heat on medium low (don't let the pan overheat). Place the apple slices in the pan and cook, turning often, for 10 to 12 minutes (depending on how thin your slices are), until they are soft enough to break with a fork or spatula.

Cover the apple slices with the brown sugar and water. Cook for 2 to 3 minutes longer, until the apples are the consistency that you would like. Remove from heat and serve.

Per serving: 95 calories, 1 gram protein, 26 grams carbohydrates, 0 gram fat, 4 grams fiber, 2 milligrams sodium

Skinny Caramel and Peanut Butter Apple

You won't believe that this treat is allowed on your diet. Whip up multiple servings to take to your next party or girls' night.

MELT ONLY

Makes 1 serving

- 2 ounces whipped fat-free cream cheese
- ½ teaspoon sugar-free caramel (coffee) syrup
- 1 teaspoon low-fat peanut butter
- 2 packs (1 teaspoon) Splenda sugar substitute
- 1 medium apple, cored and sliced

Place the cream cheese in a small bowl. Stir in the caramel syrup, peanut butter, and sugar substitute. Mix well. Serve alongside the apple slices.

Per serving (includes apple and dip): 184 calories, 10 grams protein, 34 grams carbohydrates, 2 grams fat, 7 grams fiber, 445 milligrams sodium

Skinny Fruit Dip

MELT
ONLY

This creamy dip is scrumptious when served on top of Skinny Brown Sugar Apples (page 152) or with fresh apple slices, strawberries, or melon. Seriously, it's amazing!

Makes 1 serving

2 ounces (or ¼ cup) whipped
fat-free cream cheese

¼ teaspoon vanilla extract

2 packets (1 teaspoon) Splenda
sugar substitute

Place the cream cheese in a small bowl. Stir in the vanilla and sugar substitute. Mix well. Cover and refrigerate or serve right away.

Note: *Calorie count is for fruit dip only. You will need to add in calories for any fruit you use.*

Per serving: 61 calories, 8 grams protein, 6 grams carbohydrates, 0 gram fat, 2 grams fiber, 400 milligrams sodium

Skinny Death by Chocolate

This dessert is sure to please lovers of white and milk chocolate alike. It's quick and easy to make. Enjoy it for an afternoon pick-me-up or save for a nighttime "Gotta have my chocolate" fix.

IGNITE
and
MELT

Makes 4 servings

1 box (1 ounce) Jell-O Fat-Free Sugar-Free White Chocolate Instant Pudding

2 cups fat-free milk

½ tablespoon semisweet chocolate chips

Follow the 5-minute pudding directions on the box. After the pudding has set, measure out ½ cup in a serving dish and sprinkle with the chocolate chips.

Per serving: 73 calories, 4 grams protein, 13 grams carbohydrates, 0 gram fat, 0 gram fiber, 355 milligrams sodium

Skinny Jeans
ROCK ST☆R

Before: Size 8   After: Size 6

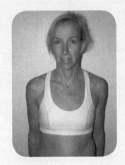

Name: Anne

Age: 43

Occupation: Mom

Children: 2

Pounds lost: 5.7

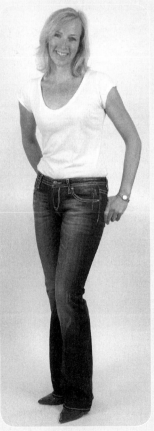

What I was afraid of: Being able to stick with the program while feeding my family.

What I liked: The results! I also never felt hungry and liked the workouts, too, especially the stretching routine.

What I learned: The program works! And it wasn't difficult to make foods for me that the family enjoyed, too.

What I want to share: I'd encourage anyone wanting to make changes to her physique to follow the Skinny Jeans program faithfully. She will not be disappointed with the results.

Chapter 8

Week 4: CARBS AND SANITY!

My Skinny Action Plan

☐ Restock my Skinny foods.

☐ Stay hydrated.

☐ Don't gorge on carbs.

☐ Keep up my food and exercise logs.

☐ Push the workouts a little harder.

☐ Supercharge My Skinny.

☐ Smile!

You made it through the Ignite phase!

Isn't the world a much more beautiful place? The sun is out, the birds are chirping, and you, my dear, can have fruit.

You are quickly earning your Rock Star status. If you were really struggling these last few weeks with not having fruit and starchy carbs, your entire existence is about to change. Your desire to strangle random people is going to significantly decrease. Not only are you going to start liking people again, but people are going to start liking you again, too.

That said, this isn't the end of the journey. It's not time to fall face-first into a bowl of pasta or a plate of cheese fries. Just give me 3 more weeks of wholehearted dedication, and I will give you smaller jeans.

Skinny Jeans Calendar: Week 4

D = Diet; E = Exercise; A = Attitude (food log)   SMS = Supercharge My Skinny

MON	TUE	WED	THUR	FRI	SAT	SUN
☐ **D** Melt	☐ **D** Melt	☐ **D** Melt	☐ **D** Melt	☐ **D** Melt	☐ **D** Melt	☐ **D** Melt
☐ **E** Firm	☐ **E** Burn	☐ **E** Off	☐ **E** Blast	☐ **E** Firm	☐ **E** Burn	☐ **E** Off
☐ **A** Journal	☐ **A** Journal	☐ **A** Journal	☐ **A** Journal	☐ **A** Journal	☐ **A** Journal	☐ **A** Journal
☐ SMS	☐ SMS	☐ SMS	☐ SMS	☐ SMS	☐ SMS	☐ SMS

Batten down the hatches, pull motivation from your Can-Do Society, and *rock out* these last 3 weeks!

Carbapalooza

This ain't no party. This ain't no free-for-all. And this sure as heck ain't a "No Carb Left Behind" tour. Before you make a mad dash to the pantry, remember that just because you're having carbs and fruit again, you're not quite home free.

In the past few weeks, you were able to eat and eat and eat some more and still had a hard time hitting your calories. But remember, that was because the veggies and protein you were eating weren't really calorie dense. When you start adding heavier foods back into your diet, you will need to be even *more* mindful of what you're putting into your mouth, and *super* diligent in writing it down. I know. It's a trade-off. But if you're not careful, you will gain back that weight and those inches. Remember: Calories in, calories out!

As we move into the Melt phase, go back and refresh your memory on what your Melt plate will look like (page 122). Don't wait! Look at your Melt plate now. That's what your next 3 weeks will look like. Memorize it. Own it.

It's also important to keep what you learned during the first 3 weeks at the forefront of your mind, because those were the weeks that helped break any sugar, junk food, or alcohol addictions you might have had. Replacing those indulgences with more nutritious options should have helped cut out your cravings. But be warned: If you just throw caution to the wind, you'll easily find yourself back in your old habits *and* your old jeans!

Don't do it! Stay the course!

Drive on By

Drive-thru dining isn't just *fast food* in the sense that it's quick and easy to get on the road; it's also fast because as soon as you eat it, it goes speeding right to your butt!

I'm not going to lie to you. I absolutely love Burger King's french fries. However, if you want to get into—and *stay in*—your skinny jeans, don't even *think* about putting that junk in your body.

The Evil Trainer in me says, "If you so much as consider grabbing fast food during these 6 weeks, I'm going to come to your house and personally kick your butt."

The Cheerleader in me, however, understands that sometimes it might be your one and only option.

So if—and only if—you are faced with dying of starvation, I'm going to tell you how to get drive-thru without derailing your diet.

Drive Through . . . If You *Have* To . . .

Do *not* supersize anything.

Ditch the bun.

Ditch the fries.

Order water.

Leave off the sauces and mayo.

Your go-to should be a garden salad with light dressing or oil and vinegar. If you like, you can opt for a salad containing grilled chicken (that is, if you honestly believe it's real chicken; I personally have my doubts).

TOP PICKS, IF YOU MUST (I'M WATCHING YOU!)

The calories for the items listed below[1] are shown without dressing. Salad dressing is the number one culprit for making your salad high in fat and calories; see My Big Fat Salad (page 203). With that said, if you absolutely *must* have dressing, ask for a light dressing or, better yet, olive oil and vinegar if the restaurant offers it.

Subway: Veggie Delite Salad
No dressing
50 calories, 9 grams carbohydrates, 1 gram fat

Subway: Turkey Breast Salad
No dressing
110 calories, 11 grams carbohydrates, 2 grams fat

Wendy's: Garden Side Salad
Light ranch dressing
70 calories, 7 grams carbohydrates, 5 grams fat

McDonald's: Side Salad (no croutons)
Newman's Own Low Fat Family Recipe Italian Dressing (1 packet: 1.5 ounces)
80 calories, 12 grams carbohydrates, 0 gram fat

Burger King: Garden Salad (values include croutons—which you will *not* eat!)
No dressing
70 calories, 7 grams carbohydrates, 4 grams fat

STAYING OUT OF THE DRIVE-THRU LANE!

Carry bags of nuts (watch the amount; these are high in calories and fat).

Keep a bottle of water in your car. Hydrating properly will keep you fuller longer!

Stash sugar-free gum in your glove compartment to keep your mouth busy!

Be totally prepared before you hit the road, and bring a cooler with you that's packed with healthy food!

How to Stay on the Wagon (Without Going Postal)

Let's face it: If you're a drinker of any kind—from a lightweight to a hard hitter—not having the grain and the grape can be a little tough. With my too-real-for-reality-TV life, there are plenty of situations that call for a good, stiff drink. But hey, you've made it to week 4 without the stuff, so another couple of weeks won't kill you. Right?

Keeping It Together

Drink sparkling water from a wine glass or beer mug. LaCroix has become my new best friend!

Fill your fridge with bottles and/or cans of sugar-free drinks like water, sparkling water or seltzer, sugar-free Crystal Light, and diet soda (limit diet soda, however; it is packed with chemicals). When you feel like popping a top or a cork, pull out one of those puppies.

Avoid the liquor store and the beer aisle of the market altogether. You might take a hostage!

Give Me Coffee or Give Me Death!

On to another addictive beverage of choice: coffee. There has been so much written and said about the pros and cons of caffeine. You will hear that caffeine is the best new thing for memory, metabolism, and weight loss. Then 5 minutes later, there will be breaking news that caffeine will kill you. Oh, the joys of scientific research! If you try to keep up with it, you'll drive yourself crazy! So I'm just going to give you my five cents as a lover of caffeine.

When I'm without my caffeine, I'm like the Hulk: big, green, and mean! Does that mean I might be slightly addicted to it? Maybe, but at some point we have to be human and give ourselves a break. I believe that coffee is the lesser evil of other things I could be addicted to. If it keeps my head from spinning and pea soup from flying out of my mouth, then so be it.

Note that I'm just talking brewed black coffee here. I'm not giving you a green light to drink a huge frozen mocha cappuccino for your caffeine fix. There is a humongous difference between a 2-calorie black coffee and an up-to-600-calorie drink filled with sugar. Stick to black coffee or coffee with skim milk and a little bit of calorie-free sweetener like Splenda or Truvia. And since java is a diuretic, make sure you drink an extra 8-ounce glass of water to compensate for each steaming cup.

Make Exercise Fun

Have you ever heard the expression *skinny fat?* If not, allow me to enlighten you, because if you don't exercise while dieting, it's exactly what you'll be called. "Skinny fat" people *look* skinny, but they have a high level of body fat and zero muscle tone. You want to be toned because the more beautiful lean muscle you have, the faster your metabolism will speed along, and the quicker you'll lose weight and keep it off.

If you've been really struggling to get through your workouts these past few weeks and not taking advantage of opportunities to make Supercharge My Skinny work for you, it's time for an attitude adjustment. By making some simple changes to your routine and to the way you view exercise, you may actually learn to thoroughly enjoy working up a sweat!

Psych Out Your Workout

Make a conscious effort to put a positive spin on the words and feelings you have toward exercise (see Chapter 2, page 31).

Turn on the tunes. Fill up your iPod with music that motivates you and puts you in a happy place. Music not only will make you want to move but also will help the time go by faster.

If you haven't done so yet, sucker your friends into exercising with you. I'm a master at this! Everything is more fun when you have someone to laugh with.

Change up (or find some) Supercharge My Skinny activities. There are probably a bunch of calorie-burning activities you enjoy that I haven't mentioned. So get creative!

Change the time of day when you exercise. If working out early in the morning is getting monotonous, work out later or vice versa.

Play! Yes, play. You have kids? Run around and kick the soccer ball or shoot hoops with them. Don't have kids? Try to remember what it was like to be one. You didn't ride a bike because you had to; you did it because it was fun! Try to look at exercise with this mentality.

Take it outside. There's nothing that makes me happier than a nice breeze and fresh air. This is especially true if you're stuck inside a stuffy office all day. Walk, jog, bike, or jump rope outside and see how much your mood will change.

Sign up for a 5-K (or 10-K!) walk or run that benefits a charitable organization. You will be helping yourself out by helping others. It's a beautiful thing.

Set playful goals for yourself. For example, put away $5 for every Skinny Jeans workout you get through. Keep that money tucked away, and at the end of your 6-week journey, take that money to buy a (nonedible) reward like a new outfit or a spa date.

When all else fails, suck it up, stop complaining, and just do it anyway. You have your skinny jeans to look forward to!

Supercharge My Skinny!

Just Put One Foot in Front of the Other!

To tell you the truth, I haven't always been a fan of running. In fact, I still don't actually *like* going for a jog or hitting the treadmill (but I'm slowly changing my perspective). If I don't *like* it, why do I keep at it, you ask? I love what it does for my body. And when I allow myself to get past the uncomfortable stage(s), it becomes almost Zen-like. If you'll give it a try, you'll learn to love the upsides, too.

Running gives you a major calorie-burning bang for your buck, and because you can do it anywhere with no equipment, it's really a superefficient way to get in a workout.

If you are new to running, start by alternating jogging and walking briskly. Begin with a four-to-one interval (4 minutes walking briskly, 1 minute of jogging). As you build strength and stamina, you can increase the jogging interval. Soon, running for 20 minutes will be easy.

Here are a few ways to make the superburn a little sweeter.

Grab a friend. You may be so out of breath that you can't talk, but you can still exchange supportive glances from time to time and chat while stretching and cooling down.

Bring your favorite tunes. Cue up your highest-energy music and run to the beat.

Take the scenic route. Head over to your local greenway or park or just the sidewalks of a beautiful neighborhood. If you live in a city, there is probably a river or some landmarks for you to jog by. Running is a great way to see the sights!

Try the "next one" technique. Look for a landmark—such as a building, an electric pole, or a tree—in the distance and keep running until you hit it. Tell yourself, "Okay, I'm going to keep going until I hit the next _____." This is a great mind game that will push you farther without your even realizing it.

You can do the same with your music. Tell yourself, "I'm going to run one more song. I made it through this one; I can make it through one more." It really works!

What You Need to Know Before You Go

Read back over Take It Outside (page 63), and make sure you're geared up with comfortable, moisture-wicking clothing and a good pair of running sneakers. And be sure to hydrate before and after you hit the road. Most researchers suggest that you consume 8 ounces of water 30 minutes before exercising and then another 8 ounces for every 15 to 20 minutes that you are at it. So if you are going for a long run on a hot day, take water with you! After the run, try a smartwater—an enhanced water that contains electrolytes without the added sugar of sports drinks.

Never Say Die

If you want to win at this fitness thing—and in the game of life in general—you have to learn to overcome obstacles and setbacks. You can't give up or give in every time something doesn't go your way.

What does this have to do with a diet program? Everything! If you dive into a cheesecake every time you have a moment of weakness, you're going to fail. You can't eat crap without looking crappy. Remember—that's the kind of behavior that led to those fat jeans to begin with.

I don't want you to cheat at all. I don't even want you to eat a piece of cake at your best friend's wedding. But if you do, *for the love of all that's holy*, don't keep shoveling it! Don't take a small mistake and turn it into a huge setback! If you fall off the wagon, don't use it as an excuse to pitch a tent and stay there for the night!

Sometimes all it takes is the tip of one domino to set off a

> "*Fall down seven times, get up eight.*"
> —Japanese proverb

chain reaction, and the whole line topples. It starts with an innocent slice of cake, and then it turns into a glass (or three) of wine. Now you're feeling guilty *and* loopy. So you say to yourself, "What the heck. I've already blown it; I might as well have a good time!" Next thing you know, you're throwing elbows at the buffet line. *Don't do it!*

A word from the Evil Trainer: "You can't throw in the towel every time you screw up your diet, so don't screw up! If you don't give in to temptation, you won't have anything to worry about!"

A word from the Cheerleader: "However, if you do happen to mess up, just stop. Forgive yourself immediately, and don't go any further. You are stronger than any temptation. Walk away from the table!"

If you're going to wear those skinny jeans, you've got to be consistent and show restraint with your eating habits.

According to Jack Canfield, one of my favorite authors, persistence is the quality that high achievers are most likely to have in common. They don't give up when the going gets tough. And they get back up when they fall.

Right now you have a choice. You can either be part of the Failed Diets Club or be a part of Jack's High Achievers Club. Which is it going to be? It's totally up to you.

Be Impeccable

Remember that promise you made to yourself in Chapter 1? The one where you promised to give this program and yourself 100 percent effort? Winners are impeccable about keeping their word. You have a promise to keep!

You have to be impeccable about your consistency in eating healthy and staying active. Why? Because the more you do both on a consistent basis, the faster and more powerfully they will become habits. They will become just as much of your routine as brushing your teeth and making your bed.

On the other end of the spectrum, if you consistently dive off the deep end or dive into the entire bag of cookies every time a crumb touches your lips, that too, will become a habit—and so will your fat jeans.

Expect more of yourself. And when you fall, get back up!

Change Your Address

Watch out: I'm gonna go all self-help on you now. (You *are* reading the attitude section; what did you expect? Recipes?)

I hit on this a little bit in Make Exercise Fun (page 162), but it deserves a little more stew time. I'm sure you've heard the saying, "Possession is nine-tenths of the law." Well, I believe *perception* is nine-tenths of your success. If you don't believe it, how will you achieve it? If you think something sucks, how are you going to bring yourself around to doing it? If you constantly complain, do you really believe you're going to enjoy it? It ain't happening!

Changing your perception is such a simple concept. If you look at the world with a can-do, love-to-do spirit, there will be nothing you can't accomplish.

You've Got to Get *Uncomfortable*

We live in a comfort-filled world. We love our comfy pajamas, comfortable shoes, cushy chair, and indulgent food. It's no wonder we've become a fat, lazy society. No one really wants to be uncomfortable! But isn't that what makes us better and stronger?

For some people, exercise is very uncomfortable, and they hate every second of it. Some people would rather go to the dentist than spend an hour in the gym. If that's you, I'm sorry, but I promise that you *can* love being active! I personally believe that "comfort" and "fun" are all in our heads, simply a matter of perception. With a single change in your thought patterns, you can learn to enjoy something. I'd even say that you can learn to *love* something. And I'll take it a step further and tell you that you can desire it so strongly that you'll be upset when you're not able to experience it!

I know because I've been there.

Drink the Kool-Aid

Recently I helped a group of women train for and compete in their first triathlon. Some had never run more than a mile before we got started. Some hadn't been on a bike since they were kids. And some—myself included—had to learn how to swim. Talk about getting uncomfortable!

Do you think we all tripped up, complained, and doubted ourselves from time to time? You'd better believe it!

But when we all crossed the finish line for the first time ever, we were filled with unbelievable joy and an outstanding sense of accomplishment that made all the discomfort and setbacks worthwhile.

Skinny Fiction: Any Form of Exercise Increases Your Hunger

Though there is research that both supports and rejects this argument, I've come to believe that increased hunger after moderate workouts like the ones in this program is more mental than an actual need for food.

The issue is that many people feel that after they've worked out, they should fill back up on large quantities of food. This is no more evident than in the group fitness world. Have you ever noticed group fitness instructors who are a little on the heavier side? I know women who teach 4 hours a day and are still a good 10 to 20 pounds overweight. Why is that? In my experience, it's because they think, "Well, I just worked out really hard, so I can eat more." And they may convince themselves that they're hungry and it's okay to eat whatever they want, as much as they want.

The truth of the matter is that if you eat more calories than you burn off, you will not lose weight. End of story. Take this into consideration regardless of how exercise may alter your appetite.

My mantra to myself and to my team of ladies (we call ourselves Team TRI Pink) was "Get uncomfortable." We all learned to embrace the feelings and feedback that our bodies were giving us. And you know what? We all changed our perception about what we were doing. Most of us quickly learned to *love* swimming, biking, and running. Whether it was the fresh air, the time away from screaming kids, or how amazing we started to feel both physically and mentally, these newfound sports truly became *fun*.

When we started training, one of the women said that she hated to run and couldn't go for more than a couple of minutes without feeling like she was going to die. I can't tell you how many times I had to talk her out of giving up. But she didn't quit, and within a year of running her first mile on the treadmill with me, she ran her first half marathon at an impressive 2 hours and 13 minutes. She is now a dedicated runner and athlete for life.

I don't necessarily expect you to go out and start training for a triathlon or marathon tomorrow. My point here is that so many of these women accomplished what they *hated*, what they thought was *impossible*. And they did it all despite their initial negative thoughts and beliefs. By changing their perception, they changed their lives.

And you can, too.

Finding Your Mojo

I seem to have lost my mojo! If you're a fan of Austin Powers, you know that *mojo* refers to Powers's sexual essence, his being. (Yeah, baby!) I love that movie! But that's not the mojo I'm talking about. I'm referring to *motivation!* Everyone needs a carrot, something to work toward, something that moves them. It's the big payoff—the pot of gold at the end of the rainbow.

Earlier in my career, my mojo was knowing that I had to be on a stage in a tiny bikini being judged in front of several hundred people. If that doesn't

THE SKINNY—*From Someone Who's Been There*

"I've learned that when I feel good about my body, I feel much better about everything else in my life."
—*Carol, Skinny Jeans Rock Star (page 14)*

motivate you to get thin quick, nothing will. No one wants to see a marshmallow butt in a bikini under stage lights. Trust me, it ain't pretty!

These days, my mojo has changed. Now it's staying sexy for my husband, ensuring my own health, wellness, and vanity; and inspiring people like you.

So what's *your* mojo? What really makes your heart race with excitement when you think about it? What is so exciting or important to you that you would make a 100 percent commitment to achieve it?

Then do it *as if!*

_____

Write your mojo here. I dare you!

_____

Are you having trouble finding some mojo? Allow me to help you. Right now, make a commitment to post before and after photos of yourself on www.amycotta.com. Let the world see your progress. That makeover ought to motivate you!

How to Act "As If"

A personal-training client recently said to me, "Okay, I think I'm really ready to give it everything I've got this time. I really want to get my body back."

I think my response surprised her. "What do you mean, you 'think'?" I replied. "You're either willing to do what it takes or you're not."

She tried again. "Well . . . I think I'm ready. I really want to lose the weight, but I know me. I'll just go back to my old ways."

"Well, what would it take to make you succeed?"

She paused. "I don't know."

"Could you lose 30 pounds in 6 weeks for $1 million?" I challenged.

"Yes!"

"What if your dad said, 'Honey, I will give you $100,000 if you lose 30 pounds in 6 weeks'?"

"Yes!"

"Okay, so what's stopping you? If you know that you'll accomplish your goal with $1 million on the line, do it! Do it *as if* there's $1 million waiting for you. Besides, isn't being happy and healthy worth more than $1 million? Isn't loving yourself worth more than that?"

My same advice goes for you. Act as if.

My Skinny Check-In

☐ I restocked my Skinny foods.

☐ I stayed hydrated.

☐ I didn't gorge on carbs.

☐ I Supercharged My Skinny!

☐ I kept my food and exercise logs.

☐ I pushed the workouts a little harder this week.

☐ I smiled!

Skinny Jeans
ROCK ST★R

Before: Size 8   After: Size 6

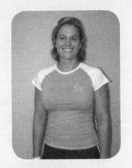

Name: Fran

Age: 39

Occupation: Mom

Children: 2

Pounds lost: 15.8

What I was afraid of: Failure

What I learned: I can do what I put my mind to! If you really work hard, it can pay off quick! Eating healthy food changes your attitude, your energy, and overall well-being. Thin feels so great!

What I liked: The program was easy to follow. Recording workouts and food was a breeze.

What I want to share: I always had the mind-set that, no matter how hard I seemed to try to lose weight, I just couldn't do it. This time I just made up my mind, once and for all! I am amazed at how well I did. For once I feel really healthy and fit. For once I feel like I can do this forever! I am so grateful!

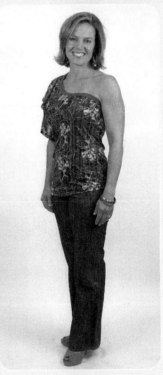

Chapter 9

Week 5: ANOTHER NOTCH ON THE BELT

My Skinny Action Plan

☐ Restock my Skinny foods.

☐ Try a harder version of some of the exercises.

☐ Supercharge My Skinny.

☐ Keep that food log going.

☐ Congratulate myself often.

Bump, bump, bump [sing with me!]
Another notch on the belt!
Da-duh, bump, bump, bump,
Another notch on the belt!
And another one's gone, and another one's gone
Another notch on the belt!

You are doing so great! Don't forget to stay in contact with me and all the other Skinny Jeans peeps on my Web site www.amycotta.com. We are there to cheer you on and help give you that last little push toward the finish line. I can't wait to see your before-and-after pictures and brag about you!

Skinny Jeans Calendar: Week 5

D = Diet; E = Exercise; A = Attitude (food log)   SMS = Supercharge My Skinny

MON	TUE	WED	THUR	FRI	SAT	SUN
☐ **D** Melt	☐ **D** Melt	☐ **D** Melt	☐ **D** Melt	☐ **D** Melt	☐ **D** Melt	☐ **D** Melt
☐ **E** Blast	☐ **E** Firm	☐ **E** Burn	☐ **E** Off	☐ **E** Blast	☐ **E** Firm	☐ **E** Burn
☐ **A** Journal	☐ **A** Journal	☐ **A** Journal	☐ **A** Journal	☐ **A** Journal	☐ **A** Journal	☐ **A** Journal
☐ SMS	☐ SMS	☐ SMS	☐ SMS	☐ SMS	☐ SMS	☐ SMS

Wok That Body!

I love Chinese food: crispy, battered meat; white rice; sugary sauces. Raise your hand if you like sweet-and-sour chicken! Unfortunately, however, this Americanized take-out favorite, usually served in astronomical portions, likes to hang around for a while . . . on my body. I might as well just glue those cute little take-out boxes to my butt and thighs.

To put it into numbers, at one popular Asian take-out spot, a serving of Orange Chicken with a side of fried rice piles up 970 calories and 38 grams of fat! Even the Eggplant Tofu with steamed rice (healthy choice, right?) adds up to 730 calories and—sit down, now—24 grams of fat.[1] Assuming that you do want more than one meal a day and don't want to slather your arteries in fat, how can you have your Chinese and eat it, too?

Real, homemade Asian-inspired food can actually be light and very healthy, filled with fresh veggies and lean meat—and let's not forget tofu and bamboo shoots!

So take a samurai sword to all those calories by making a delicious Chinese dinner yourself. Just grab a wok, throw in some good stuff, and "chopstick" your way to skinny jeans.

Here's how:

1. Dice some lean meat, seafood, or a soy product; good options include chicken, pork tenderloin, scallops, shrimp, salmon, or tofu.

2. Chop up 2 cups of vegetables, such as broccoli florets, peppers, bean sprouts, water chestnuts, and edamame.

3. Heat a nonstick pan and add a tablespoon of oil when the pan is hot.

4. Add the vegetables and sauté for about 3 minutes.

5. Stir in the meat or fish and continue sautéing until fully cooked.

6. Flavor with low-sodium soy sauce, but avoid pre-bottled Asian dressings that will add MSG, fat, and sugar to your meal. Other great flavor choices (without the calories) are ginger, pepper, and garlic.

7. For a little added texture, try sunflower seeds or water chestnuts.

8. Add some color with red, yellow, or green bell peppers for color *and* sweetness.

9. Serve over 1 cup of cooked cabbage or brown rice.

When this dish is prepared with chicken and a mixture of broccoli, snap peas, green beans, celery, onions, mushrooms, red bell peppers, and low-sodium soy sauce, it clocks in at only 303 calories. Take that, sweet-and-sour chicken!

Get a Grip

Remember back in Week 2, when we talked about hunger and how to know if you're really hungry? Well, we're gonna take it a little deeper and talk about the monkey on your back that bites you right when life throws you for a loop. That hairy little critter is called emotional eating.

If you've torn through a gallon of Ben & Jerry's after a painful breakup, if a phone call from your mother sends you running straight for the wine refrigerator, and if a bag of M&M's is the only thing standing between you and a jail cell when your husband comes home late again, you're doing some major emotional eating. And sister, you've got to get a grip!

To help you determine whether you are truly hungry or just emotional in certain situations, I've pulled some clues from the University of Texas at Austin Counseling and Mental Health Center's Web site (http://cmhc.utexas.edu/).

Actual, physical hunger takes a while to develop. It doesn't just hit you with the snap of a finger. Emotional hunger, however, is like a starving lion. It needs food now, and it's gonna tear someone up if it doesn't get it.

If you crave a certain food and once you eat it you instantly feel better, that qualifies as emotional eating. When you're truly hungry, you don't necessarily crave *only* pizza or *only* chocolate. You're more apt to make better, healthier choices.

When your tummy is full but you still crave more, you guessed it: emotional eating.

If you feel guilty after you've eaten, yep, it's emotional. And this can cause a nasty cycle: emotion → eat → feel guilty → eat → guilt → eat . . . and on and on. Eating out of real hunger and stopping when you are full won't cause you to have a guilty meltdown.

Comfort food = Mom jeans

We all have our comfort foods: those snacks (or drinks) that give you that same sensation of a warm bath or a quiet room. They help you feel like you can breathe again.

My comfort foods used to be beer and chocolate. With my "Real Housewives" life, half a bag of Dove chocolates washed back with a bottle of Miller Lite become my personal Prozac, and my indulgence led me straight to beer-gut city.

I've learned the hard way that you can't always eat what satisfies you the most. Sometimes you have to make the hard choices, and while those choices may come with an immediate sacrifice, the long-term rewards are worth it. If you continually take the easy way out, repeatedly choose the comfortable, indulgent route, you won't be rocking anything but mom jeans. If you can forgo the comfort and temptation of the here and now, your future will find you pretty comfortable in a sexy pair of skinny jeans.

"Aha!"

During my own Skinny Jeans journey, I had a major aha moment. One night when all hell was breaking loose in my house, I found myself walking out to the garage to get something to drink. Normally the fridge has beer in it, but since I had cleared the house of any and all traces of beer, I found myself popping open a can of carbonated water. I took a big swig and felt immediately better! That's when the lightbulb went off: It wasn't the beer I was craving; it was the act of walking out there, popping the can, and feeling the cold fizzy liquid on my tongue.

That moment changed everything for me. I now keep that refrigerator amply stocked with LaCroix sparkling water. My mind is happy, and the beer gut is gone. I've also learned to satisfy my chocolate craving with fruit. And I have to say, having tasted chocolate and beer a few times recently, they've both kind of lost their luster for me.

Battling the Emotional Demons

If you become more mindful of your habits and start taking stock of your emotions the way I did, you may end up having your own aha moment that will change your body and your life. Meanwhile, here are a few tips to help you take conscious control of your emotional eating habits.

As you look back over your food log from the past few weeks, you should be able to see if you were eating out of hunger or emotions. What does your hunger level tell you when compared with what you were eating?

After you've begun to recognize the times when emotional eating occurs, try to take stock of what is triggering it. Is it the screaming kids or a bad day at work? Make a list of the things that send you diving headfirst into the refrigerator.

Once you know what your triggers are, look for an alternative. My alternative was sparkling water. You can also find something productive to do instead. I became a house-cleaning, laundry-folding machine during my 6 weeks. Don't want to do household chores? Go for a walk, wash the car, or call your best friend to catch up: Do whatever you need to do to take your mind off the craving.

Learn to Love It

Okay, I'll admit it. I'm in love with exercise again. Chocolate and beer ain't got nothing on the endorphin rush I get from a good workout. And just like any other love affair, I'm cranky when I don't get to spend quality time with it.

You should know that exercise makes a really great lover. Your body was designed to need exercise and also has a built-in reward system to keep you at it! In addition to the obvious health benefits, exercise shoots your body with a dose of endorphins that make you happier and more energetic. Over time, a regular flow of those endorphins can change your attitude, your health, and quite literally your life!

So how do you fall in love? I hope you've already started! The more you exercise, the more you'll *want* to exercise. And for once, you'll have created a habit that you won't want to kick. Or, I should say, you'll have a lover you won't want to kick out.

How to Fall in Love

As with establishing any routine, you just have to set a time and do it. Write it on the calendar. Set your alarm to remind yourself if you have to. Don't make excuses. Just show up and let your body do the rest.

If you've been sticking to your exercise plan, you should already be well on your way to a serious relationship. Your body should be feeling the benefits, and as you continue to get used to regular doses of exercise and endorphins, you just won't be happy without it!

Variety Is the Spice of Life

To keep your Supercharge My Skinny and rest-day activities from becoming, well, *routine*, mix them up a bit. When the stationary bike becomes boring, try racquetball with a friend or a weekend hike. Got kids? Do double duty by riding bikes in the park or just chasing them around the backyard. Be creative. An interesting workout can make it seem less like *work* and more like going *out*.

(Also see You've Got 'Em! Burn 'Em! on page 206.)

"Oh, My Aching _____!"

The Skinny Jeans workout plans were designed to be fast, fun, and effective, and as you have probably noticed, they get progressively harder as the weeks move forward. So if you are working the plan exactly as I have mapped it out for you, you should be having one huge pain in your behind! And your legs! And the rest of your thousand and one parts!

There are actually different types of soreness. There's your normal achy kind of soreness, and then there's the "Holy cow, my legs are on fire!" soreness that almost keeps you from sitting on the toilet. That intense pain is called delayed onset muscle soreness (DOMS) and is caused by microscopic tearing in the muscle fibers. DOMS usually sets in a couple of days after a really hard workout or after you try to do something completely new at an "I've been doing it my whole life" pace.

Don't panic! DOMS is completely normal and is part of the body's natural adaptive system. Put simply, it leads to better muscle stamina and strength as the muscle recovers.

I'm sorry to say that there isn't one magic pill to cure DOMS. But here are some ways that I've found work best in both preventing and treating it.

Prevention

- **Warm up!** I can't emphasize this enough: You have got to warm up before exercise. Not only will it help offset muscle soreness, but it can also help prevent injury. I've included a warmup for you on page 74 in Chapter 5—use it!

- **Cool down!** The Daily Lube, page 112, is there for a reason.

- **Take it easy.** Don't go balls out with any new exercise or with one you haven't done in a while. Don't run 5 miles if you've barely walked 1. Gradually work up to it. And don't start back at anything as if you've never missed a day. Give your muscles a fighting chance.

- **Stick with the program.** Keep moving! A merry-go-round routine of starting and stopping and then restarting like a maniac will increase your risk of DOMS.

Treatment

Even if you give your workouts a perfect performance, you'll probably still have to deal with DOMS at some point. Try these methods for some relief.

- **Bite the hair of the dog that bit you.** A cold, tight muscle will stay that way if you don't move. The best thing you can do for yourself is *move*. Even if it hurts, move! Do something, anything, that puts those muscles in motion again.

- **Use RICE.** Don't get excited. It's not the rice you eat, but an acronym for rest, ice, compression, and elevation.

  - **Rest.** Yes, I realize I just told you to move. What I mean by *rest* is don't try doing a 5-mile run when DOMS is in full force. Use your common sense and take it a little easier than usual.

  - **Apply ice.** Put an ice pack or bag of frozen peas on the affected area, but for no more than 15 minutes at a time.

  - **Use compression.** Wrap the area comfortably in an Ace bandage before you walk or work out. If it feels too tight, it probably is. Just rewrap until it's comfortably providing compression.

  - **Elevate.** Pretty self-explanatory, huh? When you're in bed or just relaxing for the night, prop up the affected area.

- **Massage.** Ah . . . or should I say, *ouch!* When you've got a case of the DOMS, a gentle, soothing massage may hurt like hell, but it will get needed blood into your muscles to help them heal. So if you can stand it, rub yourself down or have someone else do it for you.

- **Take a yoga class.** A study done at Springfield College in Massachusetts suggests that yoga may reduce the pain of DOMS. [2]

- **Take an over-the-counter nonsteroidal anti-inflammatory drug (NSAID)** like ibuprofen (such as Advil) or naproxen (such as Aleve). This will help to temporarily reduce the soreness.

Supercharge My Skinny!

Say Hello to Mother Nature!

Are you getting tired of looking at concrete sidewalks and brick buildings when you go for a walk? Well, take it off-road! A nature hike might be just what the doctor ordered to motivate you to keep with the Supercharge My Skinny program. A wooded trail is one of my favorite places in the entire world to be. I don't know if it's the feeling of being connected with nature or the beautiful sights, sounds, and smells. It really is nature's playground for all of your senses.

Hiking on rough or hilly terrain is also one heck of a high-octane Supercharge My Skinny workout! Because the uneven terrain requires more energy, you'll be burning way more calories than by walking alone. A 150-pound woman could burn roughly 250 calories in 30 minutes! Not to mention, you'll be sculpting and strengthening your glutes, hamstrings, quadriceps, calves— pretty much everything you'll be squeezing into those jeans.

Want even more of a challenge? Pick up the pace, or try hiking with a lightly weighted back pack.

If you already know a great place to go, head over for the day! If not, just Google "hiking trails." Chances are there's a great one close to you.

What You Need to Know Before You Go

Make sure someone knows where (and the time) you are going. I like to hike with my cell phone and emergency whistle. Better safe than sorry. Make sure you have a good, sturdy pair of sneakers or hiking boots (depending on the terrain). If it is summer, spray yourself down with bug spray and sunscreen. Take plenty of water, and keep a first-aid kit in your car, just in case.

Mean Girls

Have you noticed anything different in the people around you over the last several weeks? Your family, co-workers, friends? Have they all been the supportive rock you've needed? Or have you noticed one or two of them who don't quite seem happy for you or impressed with your new life? If you haven't noticed the shift yet, just wait. It's probably coming.

Remember our Can-Do Society? You built one, right? And aren't you glad you did? The more people you have around you working with you, the better.

MEN EAT THEIR WEAK; WOMEN EAT THEIR STRONG

If I had a dollar for every dagger I've pulled out of my back from a vicious girlfriend, I would be rolling in it. We women are envious creatures, and when someone we are close to achieves something desirable, our self-centeredness (even cruelty) tends to come out.

Chances are that for every two supporters you have during your Skinny Jeans journey, there will be one mean girl. She may stay quiet for a while, secretly hoping that you'll give up in a week or so, but she is really hiding in the bushes, ready to pounce. She will want you to quit because your failure would make her feel better about herself. For her, your new body, health, and happiness are like a mirror reflecting everything she doesn't have the energy or determination to achieve.

But there is a downside to it that I didn't want to mention back then because I didn't want to discourage you from building that society. Let's talk about that now.

Not everyone in your Can-Do Society is necessarily going to be behind you, cheering you on. There are some members—most likely female—who might wish you ill behind your back. Or, if they're brash enough, they'll do it right to your face.

Meet the Mean Girls

These women are self-esteem bulldozers. These girls love conflict in any shape or form. They're like hungry sharks in a blood-filled tank, and they're ready to eat!

These girls are sly and will cover up their personal jabs with sarcasm and laughter. "Hey, Amy, you want some ice cream? Oh, wait, that's right, you're getting *skinny*." Insert evil laugh here.

You've heard it before, haven't you? Well, they come in all shapes and sizes.

The snake in the grass: You need to watch out for this chick. She's a saboteur! She wants you to fail like she wants to take her next breath. It's second nature to her. She may not just be shooting at your "fitness" good fortune; she may want to poison *every* area of your life. This chick will bring your favorite cookies to work and say, "Just take one bite. It won't kill you." She'll call you up: "Let's go out for drinks. Surely one drink won't make you fat." Do you see how she's baiting you?

The two-faced talker: This girl loves to talk out of both sides of her face. You'll get the nice one to your face: "Oh, you're doing so awesome. You look wonderful." Then her evil twin blows in right as you blow out, and she'll turn to the girl beside her and say, "Did you see her? She doesn't look like she's lost a single pound. What is she thinking?"

Granted, not knowing what she says probably won't hurt you. But let's face it: Women like to gossip. Eventually, everything that the two-faced talker said about you will make its way back around. And when it does, it's going to sting.

Storm talkers: Storm talkers don't really mean you any harm. They live on planet negative, and they can't help themselves. They will say, "You're going running? Oh my gosh, it's Saturday! I could never run. Come shopping with me instead."

Weathering the Storm

Don't hang out with negative people. It really is that simple. I've learned the hard way that the best thing you can do is put mileage between you and the haters. If someone isn't a positive light in my life, I don't have time for them. Surround yourself with people who lift you up, and ditch the ones who drag you down!

Prove them wrong! There is an old saying, "The best revenge is to live a successful life." Use the words of the mean girls as fuel for your fire. Take their negativity and make it the drive behind your every move. Go out there and prove them wrong! Do exactly what they say you cannot do!

Shake it off. If you really love the person who is being a Debbie Downer, forgive her and shake it off. She may have good intentions but just not know how to express herself. If you feel secure enough in your relationship, speak up. Tell her how her actions or words are making you feel. It just might be enough to wake her up and transform her into your biggest fan.

Sleeping with the Enemy

Your hater could also end up being the person with whom you share your bed. Oh, yes. I've had countless clients whose husbands would bring them cakes, ice cream, chocolates—you name it—while they were working hard to lose weight. Some of the men did it maliciously; some did not.

When it comes to this type of diet sabotage, there are two types of mean men in the world: the aggressive and the clueless. The aggressive ones will talk negatively toward you and about you just to make themselves feel better. The clueless ones, on the other hand, don't realize what they're doing.

If you have one of these unsupportive husbands or boyfriends, take a breath before you box him up and ship him out. Step back and have an honest look at him. Is he being mean or is he just ignorant? Men are certainly not mind readers. They're more like horses: You have to lead them to water. Tell your partner exactly what you need from him. Give him exact directions! If he's a smart horse, he'll drink the lake dry and make you a happy girl!

You've Got to See It to Believe It

I'm sure that at some point in your life, you've heard or read about visualization. It is a tool that top athletes and other high achievers use: the art of creating vivid pictures in your mind and believing in them to prepare yourself for success. Researchers have said that your brain cannot distinguish between what you're really doing and what you are only imagining doing.

What does this have to do with skinny jeans? Everything! Your body can achieve only what your mind can conceive.

Here is my very unscientific explanation. Visualization is a means of retraining your mind from "I can't" to "I already have." It's the art of tricking your mind into believing that what you *want to be* is *what you are*.

Let's say you are visualizing yourself in the mirror 20 pounds lighter in a sexy little cocktail dress. That dress may not fit you at this moment, but you are acting as if it does, you are seeing yourself in it, and you are feeling the joy and confidence that come from wearing it. Your mind believes that these pictures are real, and you must act in real life to make this visualized self come true.

I have personally used visualization to help my performance during sporting events and to lose weight and regain my body after giving birth. While I was pregnant with my second child, I used visualization

SKINNY 411
You would have to walk .04 miles to burn off one M&M's candy. Um . . . no chocolate tastes *that* good.

Skinny Fiction: Muscle Weighs More Than Fat

I'm sure at some point you've heard someone say, "Muscle weighs more than fat."

Really? One pound of muscle weighs more than a pound of fat? Don't they both weigh exactly 1 pound (16 ounces)? Let me assure you that a pound of anything is a still that: a pound. It's like saying 10 pounds of bricks are heavier than 10 pounds of feathers. They weigh the same—they just look completely different.

To my dismay, "Muscle weighs more than fat" is a widely accepted myth. Or should I say a misconception—one that some fitness professionals pass on to their clients. With this type of misinformation out there, it's no wonder why women who live and die by the scale are afraid to put on an ounce of lean muscle.

So why do so many people buy into this myth? Let me try to explain it to you this way. If you were to take two equal-size containers, filling both of them to the top—one with muscle, the other with fat—it is true that the container with muscle would weigh more. This is because muscle is 20 percent denser (it takes up less space), so more of it would fit. Fat, on the other hand, is not dense; it's fluffy and takes up mega space. Therefore, you can't fill the fat container with a portion that's equal to (as in, the same weight as) the muscle container.

Here's another visual for you—hopefully one that will help you fall in love with strength training (muscle building). Picture a big 1-pound steak and a 1-pound lump of fat. The steak is strong and sleek looking. The fat, on the other hand, is fluffy, bubbly, and gross.

This is why, when you exercise, you look slimmer and fit into smaller jeans without seeing the numbers on the scale drop. If it comes down to a choice between a smaller number on the scale and a smaller number inside my jeans, honey, I'm taking the smaller jean size any day of the week! And you should, too!

every night before going to sleep. I had committed to doing a fitness competition before finding out I was pregnant, and I knew I had only a matter of months between giving birth and standing onstage in a bikini, being judged by my peers. As I lay in bed every night, I would envision myself slim and completely fit, with no baby weight. I experienced in my mind's eye the feelings

> ## THE SKINNY—*From Someone Who's Been There*
>
> *"Before starting Six Weeks to Skinny Jeans, I bought two size 9 jeans from the juniors department. They were a little tight, but I thought, 'This will give me motivation to lose weight.' I tried them on after 6 weeks: They don't fit! The jeans don't fit because they are too big!"*
> —*Itzel, Skinny Jeans Rock Star (page 33)*

that would come with doing well in the competition and knowing that I looked great. I saw myself standing onstage and heard the announcer calling out my name as the winner.

I didn't end up winning the actual competition, but I did place fifth out of 169 women. And I'm guessing that not many of them had given birth just 4 months earlier. By regularly visualizing my goal, I had no choice but to follow what my mind thought was real. I mentally manifested everything I wanted to accomplish before actually accomplishing it.

Learning to Use Visualization: Homework!

Each night before you go to sleep, I want you to lie in your bed or somewhere you won't be disturbed. Let go of all the stress and worry of the day, and take a couple of slow, deep breaths, relaxing more and more with each one. Then I want you to close your eyes and imagine yourself walking up to a mirror. Stop in front of it, and starting from your feet, look yourself over. Notice every little detail of your body.

Now, here is the important part. See yourself as you want to look, as if it's already a reality. Feel the pleasure that comes along with seeing a flat, tight tummy. Notice how your body is reacting. Is your heart racing? Are you smiling? Do you feel confident? Are you proud of yourself? Take in all of these feelings. Keep looking at yourself in great detail. The more real you can make this moment, the better. Feel the floor beneath your feet. Is it cold? Is it soft?

What are you wearing? How does the material feel against your skin? The more details and emotions you can conjure, the more effective this exercise will be.

Do this visualization exercise every night, and I promise that it will inspire you to achieve all the goals you have set for yourself on this Skinny Jeans journey.

My Skinny Check-In

☐ I restocked my Skinny Jeans foods.

☐ I tried harder versions of some of the exercises.

☐ I Supercharged My Skinny!

☐ I kept my food and exercise logs going.

☐ I am heading to the nail salon right now! I earned a pampered treat.

Skinny Jeans
ROCK ST⭐R

Before: Size 14   After: Size 12

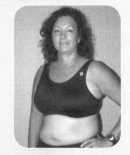

Name: Dawn

Age: 46

Occupation: Mom

Children: 2

Pounds lost: 9.6

What I was afraid of: The plan won't work. I'll be hungry. I'll get bored with the diet.

What I liked: The camaraderie among my can-do society. The exercise plans were easy to learn and didn't require special equipment. The meal plan was easy to follow. Fifteen hundred calories a day didn't sound like a lot of food, but it was!

What I learned: I have more of a sugar addiction than I thought. I also learned to eat a balanced diet through-out the day and week, to like brown rice and whole wheat pasta, to eat from the refrigerator and not the pantry, and to stop drinking soda.

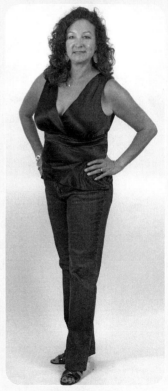

Chapter 10

Week 6: HEY, WHERE'D MY BELLY AND THIGHS GO?

My Skinny Action Plan

☐ Restock my Skinny foods.

☐ Try the hardest version of every workout.

☐ Keep logging.

☐ Go back through my log and see how successful I've been!

☐ Congratulate myself—I'm almost done!

The finish line is in sight, and look! You are skinnier! This is it. It's the final push. So *push!* Run to that finish line like you're in the Olympics!

At this point you're an old pro at this healthy-lifestyle thing. Continue to keep a watchful eye on sneaky calories, and keep writing down everything that goes into your mouth!

If you're not getting muscle tenderness anymore, your body has become accustomed to the workouts. Continue to turn up the heat and challenge yourself. Add weights or resistance bands where they aren't required. Add an extra Supercharge My Skinny workout. Make the sessions longer or more intense. Your work here isn't quite done yet, so don't exercise the same as usual. Make that little body burn! Turn on the turbocharger and disintegrate that last bit of stubborn fat!

Skinny Jeans Calendar: Week 6

D = Diet; E = Exercise; A = Attitude (food log)   SMS = Supercharge My Skinny

MON	TUE	WED	THUR	FRI	SAT	SUN
☐ **D** Melt	☐ **D** Melt	☐ **D** Melt	☐ **D** Melt	☐ **D** Melt	☐ **D** Melt	☐ **D** Melt
☐ **E** Off	☐ **E** Blast	☐ **E** Firm	☐ **E** Burn	☐ **E** Off	☐ **E** Blast	☐ **E** Firm
☐ **A** Journal	☐ **A** Journal	☐ **A** Journal	☐ **A** Journal	☐ **A** Journal	☐ **A** Journal	☐ **A** Journal
☐ SMS	☐ SMS	☐ SMS	☐ SMS	☐ SMS	☐ SMS	☐ SMS

Staying Thin While Dining In

Cooking and eating at home is always safer for your waistline than dining out because you know exactly what's going into your food. Even still, here are a few tips that could make a big difference to your diet when you're chowing down at home:

- Use a small plate and small utensils. Your portions of food will look larger, and you will take smaller bites.

- Stick to your Melt plate (see the diagram on page 122).

- Drink regular or sparkling water. If you need flavor, add a sugar-free powder mix or, better yet, squeeze in a piece of lemon or lime.

- Stop when you are full. Put extra food in the fridge or freezer for a later meal.

- Eat at the table, not in front of the TV or computer! You should be concentrating on what you are eating, not mindlessly putting food into your mouth while otherwise distracted.

- If you have a significant other or a family, try to eat together as much as you possibly can. When you are conversing, you will eat slower and the meal will last longer.

Every Step Counts

One of the easiest ways to burn calories is something you do every day, and it does not require equipment or a gym—just your two legs. You can burn some major calories morning, noon, or night just by being conscious of the steps you take!

Walk This Way

Make a game out of it! See how many steps you can take in 1 day or even a whole week. You don't need a pedometer for this, but if you have one, you'll be able to get a pretty accurate idea of the number of steps you're taking. If you're competitive or a number nerd, you'll love to watch the steps add up on that little device.

Before you really get started, count all your steps on a typical day. Try to beat that number the next day by 100 more steps, and keep going from there. Make it fun by setting daily goals for yourself and/or challenging your friends to see who can take the most steps. Compare pedometers at the end of the week, and award small prizes like a cute coffee mug or scented candle. Even if you're playing alone, reward yourself (without food) for meeting or exceeding your goals.

Here are some ways to get more steps into your day.

AT HOME

- Walk your dog. Don't have a dog? Borrow one. I'm sure your neighbor will love you for it!

- Play with your kids. Don't have kids? You can borrow those, too! Again, your neighbors will sing your praises.

- Save yourself some money and mow your own lawn. I have a training client who mows her neighbor's lawn for exercise. Seriously!

- Go for an afternoon or evening stroll with your significant other or by yourself to give your lungs a little TLC.

- While watching TV, walk around the living room, catch up on your ironing, do crunches—anything but just laze on the couch.

AT WORK

- When possible, walk to your co-worker's desk instead of phoning or e-mailing her. Besides, a face-to-face visit is much more personal.
- Take the stairs instead of the elevator or escalator.
- Go for a walk outside during your lunch break.

FOR FUN

- Go into town or to the mall for some window-shopping.
- Instead of inviting your friend over for a gossip session, ask her to meet you somewhere for a chatty stroll.

What other ways can you fit more steps into your day? Get creative!

Turn Off the Tube

We sometimes turn a deaf ear to this advice, don't we? When we hear the latest staggering statistic of how much TV time or screen time the average person gets per week, we think, "Those lazy bums! Good thing I don't watch that much TV!" But if you really track your hours of screen time, you may actually rank pretty close to that average person.

One study showed that if we just cut our TV time in half, we'd unintentionally burn more calories each day.[1] When we're not planted in our favorite chair for an hour, we find other (often much more productive) things to do. Housework, cooking, cleaning, gardening, running errands—these activities all burn more calories than watching television.

So try it, why don'tcha? Cut down your TV time as much as possible. If you have the technology, record your must-watch shows so that you can minimize your couch time by fast-forwarding through the commercials. And while you are sitting watching TV, do *something*. Knit, paint your nails, fold clothes—anything involving even the slightest movements is better than just sitting there. And if you get some of your responsibilities done then, you may have even more time to actually exercise later.

Supercharge My Skinny

The Fat Blaster

I saved the best for last: stairs! Don't worry; I've seen the fear come across my clients' faces at the mere mention of running stairs, but it's actually a lot of fun—not to mention a huge calorie burn.

For the best stair workout of all, head to your local high school or any recreation area that has a football stadium of some sort. Most high school tracks and football stadiums are open to the public. If yours isn't, ask the school if you can use it. If you are nowhere near or have no access to a stadium, find the longest, most open set of stairs you can use!

Trust me: This one little workout could completely change your body. Not only are you working your entire lower body, but you're also increasing your heart rate, and thus your endurance and stamina. You'll be able to perform other exercises for longer bouts of time without running out of steam.

Before Getting Started

Warm up. Jog around the stadium's track or on another level surface. Do the leg swings and knee circles in Chapter 5.

SKINNY 411

One-fourth of all bones in your body are located in your feet. *Take care of your feet so that they will take care of you.*

Use your entire body. Pump your arms as you run up the stairs, keeping your elbows in and shoulders relaxed, down away from your ears.

Keep your knees slightly bent. Your knees are your legs' shock absorbers. To avoid straining them, don't fully extend or lock them at any point during the workout.

Run on the balls of your feet. Your foot should strike the stair somewhere between the ball and midfoot. Running on just your midfoot will feel awkward and could increase your risk of injury.

> ### *Skinny Fiction:* The Best Time to Work Out Is First Thing in the Morning
>
> There's really no ideal time to exercise. Once you get into your new habit of being active, your body will let you know when it wants to work out. You'll have a feeling of pent-up energy that needs to be released. However, if you are a busy professional or a busy mom, the best time for your body might not work for your schedule, so exercise when your schedule allows for it, and your body will adapt to the times you choose.

Get motivated. Set a goal of how many flights up and down you are going to run.

Ease into it. Just like with any other workout, you shouldn't go out and try to move mountains the very first day. You can even start by walking a few flights, and increase your speed and workout time as you become more fit.

Make it harder. Try bounding and running up every other step. Run or jog—don't walk—on the way down!

Say It's So!

Though you may feel awkward about putting your hopes and dreams down on paper, written affirmations, like visualizations, are simple way to inspire personal

> ### THE **SKINNY**—*From Someone Who's Been There*
>
> *"I have accomplished so many things that I really didn't think I could accomplish in 6 short weeks! I have a whole new frame of mind—and it's a very positive one!"*
> —Fran, *Skinny Jeans Rock Star (page 172)*

action. So get out a notepad, a journal, or your daily planner and let the ink flow. Similar to visualizations, this forces our minds to automatically allow us to make the choices needed for us to one day live in that reality. Affirmations can be used in every area of your life, so by all means, apply them to anything and everything where you could use a little improvement.

When writing your affirmations:

1. Always start with the words *I am*. Your subconscious mind will take this as a command.[2]

2. Use the present tense. Write it out as if you have accomplished it and are already living it. For example: "I am loving being 124 pounds. I have never felt happier or healthier."

3. Keep it positive.

4. Keep it short and to the point, but be very specific.

5. Use powerful, active verbs ending in *-ing,* such as *expressing* and *working.* They give the image of doing it right now.[3]

6. Include at least one positive emotion or feeling, such as *happy, excited,* or *inspired.*

Homework: Grab some 3-by-5-inch cards and write one affirmation on each. Then post them throughout your house—on your refrigerator, on your bathroom mirror, on your computer—places you'll visit daily. I like to keep mine in the back of the book I'm reading, and I flip through them before I go to sleep each night and in the morning just before making my bed. However you choose to write them, post them, and read them, affirmations should become a part of your daily routine.

Here is an example of one of my current affirmations: "I am fit and healthy. I happily exercise every day. I maintain a healthy weight of 124 pounds. I make excellent food and drink choices to ensure my continued good health."

My Skinny Check-In

☐ I restocked my Skinny foods.

☐ I've tried the hardest version of every single workout.

☐ I'm logging! I'm logging!

☐ I've reviewed my log. Look how far I've come!

☐ I'm doing great. I feel great. I look great!

☐ Shared my success with my can-do society.

Skinny Jeans
ROCK ST★R

Before: Size 12   After: Size 8

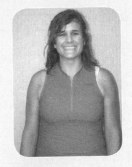

Name: Melissa

Age: 39

Occupation: Teacher

Children: None

Pounds lost: 17.4 (100 percent of weight loss was body fat!)

What I was afraid of: I was worried I wouldn't stick with the program. In the past, I had a hard time sticking to things I did on my own.

What I liked: I loved walking the journey with my friends. The Six Weeks to Skinny Jeans plan wasn't time-consuming.

What I learned: I can do it! I can do anything!

What I want to share: Never quit!

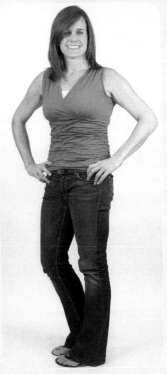

Chapter II

FROM HERE TO ETERNITY

My Skinny Action Plan

☐ Take what I have learned about health, diet, and exercise into the future. Keep the things I can live with and nix the things I can't.

☐ Don't go back to my old ways.

☐ Make exercise a way of life.

☐ Take a day off from dieting.

☐ Give this book to a friend.

☐ Live life. Love myself. Be healthy.

So Now What?

Boy, the view from here has changed! I can see that I'm now talking to a much skinnier, healthier, happier person than I was 6 weeks ago. Congratulations! And welcome to the land of skinny jeans.

That's not even the best part. This wasn't just some get-skinny-quick diet plan; this was your own personal experiment to see what eating right, exercising, and maintaining a good attitude will do for your life. And it feels pretty good, doesn't it? You are now forever equipped with the tools to stay fit and look downright sexy in *whatever* you decide to pull out of your closet.

And your journey is just beginning. You are one in a million: the one who set a weight loss goal and hit it! But don't stop there! Move the goalposts and set a new goal—a goal to *stay* skinny.

One more thing: Hang on to your fat jeans as a reminder of all that you've accomplished. And your skinny jeans? Hang them proudly in the front of your closet, where you'll see them every day.

The future is ahead of you. Don't look back!

Forever in Skinny Jeans

Since I can't hang around with you forever, I'd like to use this last chapter to equip you with some tools and guidelines that will help you stay on the skinny track from here to eternity. Eat skinny! Exercise! And keep smiling!

Going Mod

We're not talking fashion here, honey. I'm talking about *moderation*. Don't forget about the discipline you kept these past 6 weeks to get out of your fat jeans and into your skinny jeans. If you stray too far from what you've learned, I guarantee you'll end up right back where you started, or pretty darn close to it.

Now, I'm not saying you can't enjoy some of the simple things in life that bring us joy, like a cup of hot chocolate, a handful of chips, an ice-cold beer, or a slice of New York–style pizza. But if you indulge in these things too often, fail to practice portion control, and give up exercise, you will grow right back out of the skinny jeans you just busted your butt to fit into.

Portion Control

After being so disciplined for so long, a seven-layer chocolate cake may look like a pretty tempting way to celebrate. By all means, have a slice, but you know better than to dive in face-first and demolish half before that first bite even hits your stomach.

You've learned about emotional eating. You know what's in a seven-layer chocolate cake—seven layers of sugar and fat! And that won't fit into your skinny jeans, now, will it?

Here are some guidelines for sizing up healthy portions of different types of foods.

ONE SERVING OF

Meat, poultry, soy protein = one deck of cards

Fish = one checkbook

White or sweet potato = one computer mouse

Green veggies = two fists

Salad dressing, oil, mayo = one poker chip

Butter or margarine = one dice

Pancake or waffle = one CD or DVD

Peanut butter = one thumb (the length from base to tip)

Cheese = one domino or six dice

Chips, popcorn, pretzels = two handfuls

Dried fruit or nuts = one golf ball or egg

Cooked rice or pasta = one round handful

Frozen yogurt or ice cream = one tennis ball

Portion Practice

Of course you can read that list, hang it on your fridge, and memorize it like a good little girl, but it will do you absolutely no good until you put it into regular practice as you eat.

Here are some tips for doing just that.

- Use a salad plate instead of a large dinner plate. The smaller plate will make it look like more food, and believe it or not, it'll feel like it, too.

- Follow the Melt plate diagram (on page 122) and divide your plate into four sections. Put veggies in two sections, protein in one, and starch in the other.

- When possible, leave the food on the stove or the counter while you're eating. Don't put it on the table. You can also pack away any leftover food before you even sit down to eat. The bottom line: If the food's not sitting on the table, you're much less likely to nibble on it when your plate is empty.

- Do not immediately spring for seconds—no matter how much Grandma pushes them. Give your first serving time to hit your tummy, and then decide if you really are still hungry. You can always have leftovers tomorrow!

- At some point during the week, divide your snacks and desserts into sensible portions and put them in individual bags or containers. This will keep you from cracking open a box and devouring the entire thing. And remember to check the serving sizes and nutritional info on the back!

- Follow the magic rule "One and done" when eating yummy comfort foods, like slices of pizza or cookies. More than one will be no fun—for you or your skinny jeans.

- Drink plenty of water before, during, and after eating. Not only will this keep you well hydrated, but it will also help you feel full.

- Customize your servings. We have a tendency to scoop out the same amount for everyone, but your portions should be larger than a child's and smaller than a man's.

Restaurant Survival

You may have been good about preparing all of your own meals and eating at home during the program, but I'm not expecting you to be a homebody the rest of your life! I love going out on the town with friends and having someone else cook for me as much as the next person. Dining out is fine—as long as you do it right.

Here are some guidelines.

- Be sensible. Dining out doesn't mean you get to act like a pig at the trough. Eat the way you would at home—or better! Look for the healthiest food choice and request cooking adjustments where needed (for example, dressing on the side, veggies instead of french fries, no cheese).

- Stay away from menu items that are fried or breaded or that include heavy cream sauce, butter, or anything else that you know is high in saturated fat and unhealthy carbs.

- Tell the waiter you don't need a bread basket—or, if he brings one, ask him to take it away.

- Ask for water as soon as you are seated, and drink plenty throughout your meal.

- If you would like an appetizer, order a broth-based soup or a small green salad with dressing on the side.

- Stick to your Skinny Jeans RPH (Rate of Perceived Hunger) Scale. When you are satisfied or full, stop eating. Either have the food removed or ask for a take-out box. You can also have some of your food boxed as soon as you get your plate so that you are not tempted to stuff yourself.

- Skip or split the dessert.

My Big Fat Salad

Okay, you're gonna want to sit down for this one! Salads. They look healthy. They sound healthy. Most people are under the assumption that because a salad has a lot of lettuce (which has practically no calories), all salads are low in calories and fat. Au contraire to your derriere—that's not even close to being correct.

You know that drive-thru salad you ate the other day because you wanted to eat healthy? Well, it contained more than 750 calories! That's like a fat, juicy drive-thru hamburger and fries!

I wish I were joking.

The Ugly Truth!

McDonald's Premium Southwest Salad with Crispy Chicken (no dressing!)
470 calories, 38 grams carbohydrates, 20 grams fat, 12 grams sugars

VS.

McDonald's Single Cheeseburger
300 calories, 33 grams carbohydrates, 12 grams fat, 6 grams sugars

and

McDonald's Small Fries
230 calories, 29 grams carbohydrates, 11 grams fat, 0 gram sugars

Wendy's Baja Salad with Red Jalapeño Dressing
740 calories, 49 grams carbohydrates, 47 grams fat, 14 grams sugars

VS.

Wendy's Double Stack Cheeseburger
360 calories, 26 grams carbohydrates, 18 grams fat, 6 grams sugars

and

Wendy's Small Fries
320 calories, 41 grams carbohydrates, 15 grams fat, 0 gram sugars

A McDonald's salad has 20 grams of fat. A cheeseburger has 12 grams.

Taco Bell Fiesta Taco Salad
770 calories, 74 grams
carbohydrates, 42 grams fat,
8 grams sugars

VS.   **Taco Bell Grilled Chicken Burrito**
430 calories, 48 grams
carbohydrates, 18 grams fat,
2 grams sugars

Take a Break

I know I've said a thousand times how important it is to eat as healthy as possible in order to stay in your skinny jeans, but here's a new guideline: I want you to take a *diet break*. That's right—a cheat day, if you will.

Yes, I realize I've been telling you this whole time that you have to stick to the plan. Well, that was then, and this is now.

Now you've got to learn how to live the rest of your life on a plan you can live with. If that means you occasionally splurge and eat a stack of pancakes for breakfast, then do it. Just don't do it every day. This is where moderation is key. Eat what you want, within reason, once per week, and you'll never feel deprived again.

This diet break doesn't come without strings. In order to enjoy these breaks, you've got to follow a few rules. If you break the rules, you'd better pull out the fat pants, 'cause your butt is going to be right back in them.

THE RULES OF THE DIET BREAK

1. You may cheat only 1 day per week.

2. And by "1 day," I don't mean to pig out the entire day. This is *not* an opportunity to eat everything in sight. Use self-control and respect the skinny jeans.

3. On the day off, you *must* exercise! Remember: calories in, calories out.

4. Don't change your cheat day. Keep it the same day every week. This way you are less likely to cheat when it's not your actual cheat day.

5. Enjoy! (But not too much!)

You've Got 'Em! Burn 'Em!

You can burn 150 calories in any of the following ways:

COMMON CHORES

Washing and waxing a car for 45 to 60 minutes

Washing windows or floors for 45 to 60 minutes

Gardening for 30 to 45 minutes

Pushing a stroller 1.5 miles in 30 minutes

Raking leaves for 30 minutes

Walking 2 miles in 30 minutes (15 minutes per mile)

Swimming laps for 20 minutes

Shoveling snow for 15 minutes

Stair walking for 15 minutes

SPORTING ACTIVITIES

Playing volleyball for 45 to 60 minutes

Playing touch football for 45 minutes

Walking 1.5 miles in 30 minutes (20 minutes per mile)

Shooting baskets for 30 minutes

Bicycling 5 miles in 30 minutes

Dancing fast (social) for 30 minutes

Doing water aerobics for 30 minutes

Playing basketball for 15 minutes

Bicycling 4 miles in 15 minutes

Jumping rope for 15 minutes

Running 1.5 miles in 15 minutes (10 minutes per mile)[1]

The Incredible Shrinking Jeans

Look, you already know that the scale is a liar. We already know that you can weigh more and be in smaller jeans. On the flip side of that coin, you can weigh less and be in larger jeans. So if your skinny jeans are making you feel fat, well, then, you're probably packing the fat back on, and it's time for a reality check.

1. Do a throw-in-the-garbage-can scan of the kitchen, and get rid of any food demons that have snuck back in.

2. Log it. You know the drill. Food goes in the log before it goes in your mouth.

3. Get moving. Make sure that 60 minutes of exercise is on the books—in ink—for each of the next 6 days.

4. Think skinny. No eating out, drinking, skipping workouts, or making excuses.

5. Find nonfood ways to reward yourself at the end of each successful day. And remember: The ultimate reward will be feeling great in those skinny jeans again.

Beer Belly or Bikini Belly?

The choice is yours.

Wouldn't it be great if we could have our beer (or wine or cosmos) and our skinny jeans, too? Unfortunately, alcoholic beverages of all varieties are packed with calories, and even worse, the alcoholic content breaks down into acetate, which your body will process before burning any of the other calories you've stored up during the day.[2] So when you drink alcohol, not only are you downing extra calories, but you're also delaying your overall metabolism.

Since letting loose *and* staying in shape are both essential to my overall happiness, I have learned to think before I drink. Here's the 411.

- A 5-ounce glass of red or white wine will cost you around 150 calories.
- A pint of Hefeweizen (German wheat beer) clocks in at around 151 calories.
- A 6-ounce margarita will set you back 300 calories.
- A piña colada will cost you a whopping 526 calories.
- A Miller MGD 64 beer will rack up only 64 calories.

So enjoy, but be sure you make up for those calories by either eating less for dinner or exercising extra that day or the next. Something has to give somewhere. If not, the calories stay and the skinny jeans go.

Your Skinny Jeans Future

Going forward, commit to these simple rules, and you'll be happy, healthy, and rocking those skinny jeans for life!

Work out at least 20 minutes per day, no fewer than 3 days per week. And this isn't a dog walk: I mean *sweat*. Push yourself.

- Stay active every day you don't officially work out. Take the stairs; walk during lunch. Look back over You've Got 'Em! Burn 'Em! on page 206.
- Stick to the Melt eating plan as closely as possible from here on out. This means staying away from high-sugar, high-starch foods such as white potatoes, white rice, and pasta, and of course fried food and junky snacks. Eat plenty of high-quality, fiber-filled veggies, whole grains, and lean proteins.
- Unless it's your cheat day, limit or avoid fried food, fast food, or anything overly packaged and processed.
- Try not to eat out more than once per week, and don't overindulge when you do.
- Drink eight full 8-ounce glasses per day. Keep a water bottle with you at all times.

- Try to limit your alcohol consumption to 1 night per week. Follow the moderation rules.

- Keep those skinny jeans handy, and put them on often. When they start feeling too tight, it's time to batten down the hatches, turn up the heat, and apply what you've learned from this book. Remember you can always walk the walk again. But you're not going to need to, because you're going to maintain your new lifestyle!

Moving On

Well, we're here. It's time to say good-bye. I hope you've enjoyed this journey as much as I've enjoyed writing it and living it. I've had so many aha moments along the way and learned a lot about the person I've become. I hope you've had some of those moments yourself. I would love it if you would share them with me at www.amycotta.com.

Keep in Mind

It's really easy to break out of your new habits and to fall back into old ones. If you find yourself doing this, remind yourself how hard you've worked to get here. Take it from me: It's much easier to maintain your health and fitness from now on than it is to start all over. If you find yourself starting to fall back into old patterns of emotional eating or drinking, stop yourself dead in your tracks. You've got to keep all those old demons at bay. Focus on the positive new you.

Also, be sure to keep up the exercise. Make fitness a lifestyle. Make it as much a part of your daily routine as brushing your teeth. You don't have to be as hardcore as you've been the last 6 weeks, but take what you've learned and mold it into something that you can easily live with.

If you find yourself in need of some encouragement or a swift kick in the pants, remember that I'm always here. Just pull me off the shelf and dust me off. I could use the exercise!

Epilogue
CROSSING OVER

I've been to the dark side, and it isn't pretty. I know what having a marshmallow booty and a potbelly feels like. I know what it's like to suffer from IUsedTo disease. I know what it feels like to feel self-conscious in a bikini. It is miserable, to say the least.

It wasn't until I was standing in my competition bikini inside the Las Vegas Ballroom at the 21st Annual Bikini America Pageant that the reality of my own Skinny Jeans journey hit me like a tidal wave. It was like coming out of a fog and being able to see clearly for the first time. I had crossed over.

There I stood, 20 pounds lighter than I was before I started the program. There I was, about to grace the stage one more time after a 6-year departure from competition. I had my body—and better yet, my self-confidence—back. I forgot how much I had missed both. I forget how much it meant to love myself.

That's when the uncontrollable tears started to fall. The tears I cried were those of joy and of anger. I cried because I was proud of myself, and I felt awesome, but I couldn't believe I had ever allowed myself to get so out of shape, to expect so little of myself, and to believe I was okay with being mediocre. I wasn't put on this Earth to be mediocre; I was put here to be exceptional, to treat my body like the temple it is.

It's a funny thing, you know, when you start to let your standards slip away. All of a sudden, what you would *never* accept for yourself becomes, "Well, I don't look *that* bad." When you let yourself go for so long, *not too fat* is okay, because at least you're not as fat as your fattest self once was. I let my standards drop, and my self-esteem was its tragic victim.

I wish I had the words to make you fully appreciate the awestruck moment I had standing there in that ballroom. Every emotion imaginable pulsated through my body. How did I allow myself to get so bad? Who was I? At what point did I lose myself? And boy, am I glad to be back!

I believe to find oneself is a true blessing. In this life you get what you accept and expect. No one can keep you trapped in mediocrity and in mom jeans except you.

Keep your standards high and you'll never cross back over to the dark side.

It truly was my greatest honor to take this journey with you. Thank you for inspiring me to remember who I am.

Live life. Love yourself. Be healthy.

Acknowledgments

I first have to thank God for putting such strong desire and passion in my heart. I'm so thankful for the drive and dreams that you entrusted me to sow. I want to spend the rest of my life praising your glory and helping to instill that light into others.

To all of my children, Kali, Tyler, Denver, Greer, Chase, and Skylar (and my grandson, Wyatt): Thank you for putting up with my hours away from you. I know it wasn't easy to share me with the computer. Thank you for allowing me to share my love for health and fitness with the world. I know I laugh a lot about how crazy our life is (and it is), but I wouldn't trade one single second of it. I love each of you with every fiber of my being. You are my heart's desire.

To my husband and best friend, Jim: God sent me an angel and a savior when you came into my life. You picked me up and breathed new life into me and my dreams. Thank you for never giving up on me. Thank you for picking up the slack when I was unable. I truly believe that the rest of our lives will be the best of our lives.

Mom and Dad: I know I wasn't always the easiest kid to deal with. But your love and understanding made me the person I am today. Thank you for your constant belief in me, even when I doubted myself. I'm so proud to call you my parents.

My team, Bill, Shawna, Stephanie, Holly: Wow! You are all so amazing! Bill, thank you for believing in me. You took a chance on a "has been" and helped turn her into a *once again*. It was that belief that motivated me to dream bigger dreams. Shawna, you are an amazing professional and friend. I don't know what I would have done without you. My dreams would have crumbled had it not been for you. I will never forget that. Stephanie, I am so blessed to have you in my life. Thank you for all your hard work and for keeping my sea calm when I was in the midst of a storm. Holly, what can I say? You rock!

My Oasis family: Thank you for guiding me back home. I was completely lost when I walked through your doors. I don't have words to express what your house and love have done for my life.

My dear friend Janet: I'm so thankful and blessed to call you friend. Thank you for always being there; you are a true gem. I love you!

Steven, Shannon, Dan, Deanna, Itzel, and Jason: Thank you all for your wonderful contributions to this book. I can't thank you enough!

Amy: This book would not have been possible without you. Had God not put you in my life, I wouldn't be typing these words right now. Thank you for your work, support, and blessings.

A special thank-you to registered dietitian Carilu Robinson for her valuable input and review of the Ignite and Melt eating plans.

To my friends and my Team TRI Pink family: You are the most amazing women (and men) I have ever had the pleasure of spending time with and sharing my love of movement with. Thank you all for your love and support over the years. Each one of you has a special place in my heart. I am a better person because of you. Remember always to *get uncomfortable* and believe in yourself.

Skinny Jean Rock Stars: Thank you for working the plan! You are all amazing. You inspired me. You are all such wonderful role models. You proved that hard work, dedication, and the right attitude pay off and pay off big! I'm so *proud* of you!

To my friends at Belle Meade Dermatology in Nashville: How can I *ever* thank you enough for erasing the years and stress from my face? Had it not been for you, a thousand hours of Photoshop would have been in order! Shona, I love you, girl!

Special thanks to Prairie Life Fitness and Meridian Fitness in Franklin, Tennessee, for allowing us to use your facilities.

Last, I would like to thank my high school principal and the rest of the naysayers and crazy people in my life. Some of you wished me ill and tried to steal my peace. God knew what he was doing when he sent you to me. You were the source of lessons that I needed to learn to get where I am today. With the most humble of hearts (I really mean this), thank you.

IGNITE AND MELT MEAL PLANS

Not sure what a day of Skinny Jeans eating looks like? Don't worry. I have assembled three daily meal plans for both the Ignite and Melt phases. Depending on your personal calorie requirements for weight loss (pages 5–6), you will need to either add or omit food to hit your caloric goals. Use these plans as a template to build your own menus, and don't be afraid to get creative. To find more recipes and foods to enjoy, come on over to www.amycotta.com. When you come up with a menu you love, please share it with the other Skinny Jeans Rock Stars. Let's take this journey together!

Ignite Days

IGNITE DAY 1

Breakfast	1 cup coffee with ¼ cup fat-free milk 2 slices Canadian bacon Egg White–Spinach Scramble: In a medium pan coated with olive oil cooking spray, wilt 2 cups spinach, then add 4 large egg whites and scramble until cooked. *Per serving: 155 calories, 31 g protein, 7 g carbohydrates, 1 g fat, 1 g fiber, 483 mg sodium*
Snack 1	½ cup sliced cucumbers 2 Mini Babybel Light cheese rounds *Per serving: 108 calories, 12 g protein, 2 g carbohydrates, 5 g fat, 0 g fiber, 321 mg sodium*
Snack 2	1 sugar-free chocolate pudding cup *Per serving: 60 calories, 2 g protein, 13 g carbohydrates, 2 g fat, 1 g fiber, 190 mg sodium*
Lunch	1 serving Skinny Colorful Salad (page 128) 4 ounces grilled chicken breast 1 piece Sargento String Cheese Part-Skim Mozzarella Cheese *Per serving: 348 calories, 44 g protein, 10 g carbohydrates, 14 g fat, 2 g fiber, 587 mg sodium*
Snack 3	½ ounce (11) almonds, dry roasted *Per serving: 85 calories, 3 g protein, 3 g carbohydrates, 8 g fat, 2 g fiber, 0 mg sodium*
Dinner	1 Skinny Beef Kebob (page 134) 2 cups baby spinach mixed with ¼ cup grape tomatoes, 2 tablespoons light feta cheese, and 1 tablespoon reduced-calorie Caesar dressing *Per serving: 413 calories, 28 g protein, 12 g carbohydrates, 28 g fat, 3 g fiber, 535 mg sodium*
Snack	1 Skinny Parfait (page 151) *Per serving: 199 calories, 17 g protein, 18 g carbohydrates, 7 g fat, 3 g fiber, 0 mg sodium*
Total calories: 1,369	

IGNITE DAY 2	IGNITE DAY 3
1 cup coffee with ¼ cup fat-free milk 3 Skinny Minis (page 132) *Per serving: 377 calories, 48 g protein, 10 g carbohydrates, 15 g fat, 0 g fiber, 1,685 mg sodium*	12 ounces coffee or tea with ¼ cup fat-free milk Egg-White Omelet: Beat 5 egg whites together in a small bowl, then pour into a medium pan coated with olive oil cooking spray. Top with ¼ cup chopped bell pepper (any color) and ¼ cup grated reduced-fat Cheddar cheese, then slide a spatula underneath and fold the omelet in half. Cook until the eggs are completely set. *Per serving: 196 calories, 28 g protein, 7 g carbohydrates, 5 g fat, 1 g fiber, 555 mg sodium*
30 peanuts, dry roasted 1 Mini Babybel Light cheese round *Per serving: 226 calories, 13 g protein, 6 g carbohydrates, 18 g fat, 2 g fiber, 162 mg sodium*	½ ounce (22) almonds, dry roasted *Per serving: 169 calories, 6 g protein, 5 g carbohydrates, 15 g fat, 3 g fiber, 0 mg sodium*
1 Sugar-Free Jell-O Pudding Cup *Per serving: 60 calories, 2 g protein, 0 g carbohydrates, 2 g fat, 1 g fiber, 190 mg sodium*	1 cup Skinny Death by Chocolate (page 155) *Per serving: 146 calories, 8 g protein, 26 g carbohydrates, 1 g fat, 0 g fiber, 710 mg sodium*
1 serving Skinny Lettuce Wraps (page 137) *Per serving: 338 calories, 50 g protein, 27 g carbohydrates, 6 g fat, 11 g fiber, 127 mg sodium*	1 serving Skinny Stuffed Red Peppers (page 133) 3 pieces Skinny Crab-Deviled Eggs (page 139) *Per serving: 453 calories, 54 g protein, 24 g carbohydrates, 15 g fat, 6 g fiber, 710 mg sodium*
2 pieces Sargento String Cheese Part-Skim Mozzarella Cheese *Per serving: 100 calories, 12 g protein, 1 g carbohydrates, 5 g fat, 0 g fiber, 200 mg sodium*	1 piece Sargento String Cheese Part-Skim Mozzarella Cheese *Per serving: 70 calories, 6 g protein, 1 g carbohydrates, 5 g fat, 0 g fiber, 200 mg sodium*
6 ounces grilled tilapia 1 serving Skinny Cucumber Salsa (page 141) 3 servings Skinny Crab-Deviled Eggs (page 139) *Per serving: 334 calories, 46 g protein, 10 g carbohydrates, 12 g fat, 3 g fiber, 303 mg sodium*	1 serving Skinny Mexican Stir-Fry (page 130), topped with 1 serving Skinny Guacamole (page 143) and ¼ cup grated reduced-fat Cheddar cheese *Per serving: 352 calories, 37 g protein, 14 g carbohydrates, 17 g fat, 5 g fiber, 558 mg sodium*
1 Skinny Ice Pop (page 150) *Per serving: 6 calories, 0 g protein, 2 g carbohydrates, 0 g fat, 0 g fiber, 5 mg sodium*	1 serving Skinny Chocolate Delight (page 149) *Per serving: 116 calories, 7 g protein, 23 g carbohydrates, 1 g fat, 1 g fiber, 211 mg sodium*
Total calories: 1,461	**Total calories: 1,502**

Melt Days

	MELT DAY 1
Breakfast	12 ounces coffee or tea with ¼ cup fat-free milk 1 serving Skinny Waffles (page 136) with 2 tablespoons reduced-sugar maple syrup 1 cup strawberries, sliced *Per serving: 312 calories, 15 g protein, 61 g carbohydrates, 3 g fat, 9 g fiber, 640 mg sodium*
Snack 1	½ cup 1% reduced-fat cottage cheese ½ cup blueberries *Per serving: 122 calories, 13 g protein, 17 g carbohydrates, 2 g fat, 2 g fiber, 421 mg sodium*
Snack 2	1 Sugar-Free Jell-O Pudding Cup *Per serving: 60 calories, 2 g protein, 13 g carbohydrates, 2 g fat, 1 g fiber, 170 mg sodium*
Lunch	1 serving Skinny Scallop Soup (page 127) 2 cups spinach mixed with ½ cup sliced cucumber, ½ cup chopped baby carrots (raw) and 2 tablespoons Skinny Blue Cheese Dressing (page 147) *Per serving: 213 calories, 24 g protein, 22 g carbohydrates, 4 g fat, 7 g fiber, 425 mg sodium*
Snack 3	1 medium apple 1 tablespoon reduced-fat, all-natural peanut butter *Per serving: 195 calories, 5 g protein, 31 g carbohydrates, 6 g fat, 5 g fiber, 62 mg sodium*
Dinner	1 serving Skinny Stroganoff (page 135) 1 serving Skinny Palm Salad (page 129) *Per serving: 417 calories, 34 g protein, 39 g carbohydrates, 16 g fat, 8 g fiber, 539 mg sodium*
Snack	1 serving Skinny Chocolate Delight (page 149) *Per serving: 116 calories, 7 g protein, 23 g carbohydrates, 1 g fat, 3 g fiber, 211 mg sodium*
	Total calories: 1,435

MELT DAY 2	MELT DAY 3
12 ounces coffee or tea with ¼ cup fat-free milk	12 ounces coffee or tea with ¼ cup fat-free milk
½ cup rolled oats (prepared with water), sweetened with 2 teaspoons sugar substitute	1 reduced-calorie whole wheat English muffin, spread with 1 tablespoon all-natural peanut butter
¾ cup berries	6 ounces fat-free, sugar-free yogurt (plain or flavored)
2 hard-boiled egg whites (yolks removed)	½ grapefruit
Per serving: 233 calories, 17 g protein, 36 g carbohydrates, 3 g fat, 6 g fiber, 142 mg sodium	*Per serving: 384 calories, 20 g protein, 66 g carbohydrates, 9 g fat, 12 g fiber, 383 mg sodium*
4 ounces deli turkey breast, sliced	1 medium peach or nectarine
2 The Laughing Cow Light Creamy Swiss Spreadable Cheese Wedges	½ cup 1% low-fat cottage cheese
Per serving: 131 calories, 18 g protein, 2 g carbohydrates, 5 g fat, 0 g fiber, 874 mg sodium	*Per serving: 141 calories, 15 g protein, 18 g carbohydrates, 2 g fat, 2 g fiber, 459 mg sodium*
1 Sugar-Free Jell-O Pudding Cup	1 Mini Babybel Light cheese round
Per serving: 60 calories, 2 g protein, 13 g carbohydrates, 2 g fat, 1 g fiber, 190 mg sodium	*Per serving: 80 calories, 5 g protein, 0 g carbohydrates, 6 g fat, 0 g fiber, 170 mg sodium*
2 servings Skinny Palm Salad (page 129), mixed with 1 medium apple, chopped	1 serving Skinny Colorful Salad (page 128), mixed with ½ ounce (11) almonds and 1 medium orange, sliced
1 serving Skinny Squash (page 140)	*Per serving: 275 calories, 7 g protein, 30 g carbohydrates, 15 g fat, 7 g fiber, 323 mg sodium*
Per serving: 297 calories, 9 g protein, 42 g carbohydrates, 14 g fat, 14 g fiber, 853 mg sodium	
1 Skinny Caramel and Peanut Butter Apple (page 153)	1 medium apple
Per serving: 184 calories, 10 g protein, 34 g carbohydrates, 2 g fat, 7 g fiber, 445 mg sodium	*Per serving: 80 calories, 0 g protein, 22 g carbohydrates, 0 g fat, 5 g fiber, 0 mg sodium*
4 ounces chicken breast, baked with 1 serving Skinny Marinade (page 145)	8 ounces beef tri-tip, broiled
2 servings Skinny Garlic Broccoli (page 142)	2 servings Skinny Garlic Broccoli (page 142)
2 servings Skinny Parmesan Artichoke Hearts (page 138)	*Per serving: 437 calories, 55 g protein, 19 g carbohydrates, 16 g fat, 6 g fiber, 348 mg sodium*
Per serving: 362 calories, 40 g protein, 33 g carbohydrates, 10 g fat, 10 g fiber, 1,986 mg sodium	
1 Skinny Parfait (page 151)	1 Skinny Ice Pop (page 150)
Per serving: 199 calories, 17 g protein, 18 g carbohydrates, 7 g fat, 3 g fiber, 0 mg sodium	*Per serving: 6 calories, 0 g protein, 2 g carbohydrates, 0 g fat, 0 g fiber, 5 mg sodium*
Total calories: 1,466	**Total calories: 1,404**

DAILY FOOD LOGS

Why food logs, you ask? Here's the low down. In order to avoid consuming more calories than your body needs as fuel , you need to look up the calorie content of everything you eat and keep a running total of the food and calories you are consuming on any given day. You are on your way to being a Skinny Jeans Rock Star and Rock Stars are obsessed with logging their meals and snacks.

So what are you waiting for? Use the following pages and get logging!

Ignite Day I

THE FOOD LOG   DATE: _____ CALORIE GOAL: _____

TIME	FOOD	CALORIES	RUNNING TOTAL	HUNGER RATING

TOTAL CALORIC INTAKE: _____

TOTAL CALORIC EXPENDITURE: _____

WATER (8 OZ): ☐ ☐ ☐ ☐ ☐ ☐ ☐ ☐

Yay me! _____

_____

_____

Ignite Day 2

THE FOOD LOG DATE: _____ CALORIE GOAL: _____

TIME	FOOD	CALORIES	RUNNING TOTAL	HUNGER RATING

TOTAL CALORIC INTAKE: _____

TOTAL CALORIC EXPENDITURE: _____

WATER (8 OZ):

Yay me! _____

_____

_____

THE FOOD LOG DATE: _____ CALORIE GOAL: _____

TIME	FOOD	CALORIES	RUNNING TOTAL	HUNGER RATING

TOTAL CALORIC INTAKE: _____

TOTAL CALORIC EXPENDITURE: _____

WATER (8 OZ):

Yay me! _____

_____

_____

Ignite Day 4

DATE: _____ CALORIE GOAL: _____

TIME	FOOD	CALORIES	RUNNING TOTAL	HUNGER RATING

TOTAL CALORIC INTAKE: _____

TOTAL CALORIC EXPENDITURE: _____

WATER (8 OZ):

Yay me! _____

_____

_____

THE FOOD LOG   DATE: _____ CALORIE GOAL: _____

TIME	FOOD	CALORIES	RUNNING TOTAL	HUNGER RATING

TOTAL CALORIC INTAKE: _____

TOTAL CALORIC EXPENDITURE: _____

WATER (8 OZ):

Yay me! _____

_____

_____

Ignite Day 6

DATE: _____ CALORIE GOAL: _____

TIME	FOOD	CALORIES	RUNNING TOTAL	HUNGER RATING

TOTAL CALORIC INTAKE: _____

TOTAL CALORIC EXPENDITURE: _____

WATER (8 OZ):

Yay me! _____

_____

_____

Ignite Day 7

THE FOOD LOG   DATE: _____ CALORIE GOAL: _____

TIME	FOOD	CALORIES	RUNNING TOTAL	HUNGER RATING

TOTAL CALORIC INTAKE: _____

TOTAL CALORIC EXPENDITURE: _____

WATER (8 OZ): ▯ ▯ ▯ ▯ ▯ ▯ ▯ ▯

Yay me! _____

_____

_____

Ignite Day 8

THE FOOD LOG DATE: _____ CALORIE GOAL: _____

TIME	FOOD	CALORIES	RUNNING TOTAL	HUNGER RATING

TOTAL CALORIC INTAKE: _____

TOTAL CALORIC EXPENDITURE: _____

WATER (8 OZ):

Yay me! _____

_____

_____

Ignite Day 9

THE FOOD LOG DATE: _____ CALORIE GOAL: _____

TIME	FOOD	CALORIES	RUNNING TOTAL	HUNGER RATING

TOTAL CALORIC INTAKE: _____

TOTAL CALORIC EXPENDITURE: _____

WATER (8 OZ):

Yay me! _____

_____

_____

Ignite Day 10

THE FOOD LOG   DATE: _____ CALORIE GOAL: _____

TIME	FOOD	CALORIES	RUNNING TOTAL	HUNGER RATING

TOTAL CALORIC INTAKE: _____

TOTAL CALORIC EXPENDITURE: _____

WATER (8 OZ):

Yay me! _____

_____

_____

Ignite Day II

THE FOOD LOG   DATE: _____   CALORIE GOAL: _____

TIME	FOOD	CALORIES	RUNNING TOTAL	HUNGER RATING

TOTAL CALORIC INTAKE: _____

TOTAL CALORIC EXPENDITURE: _____

WATER (8 OZ):

Yay me! _____

_____

_____

Ignite Day 12

THE FOOD LOG DATE: _____ CALORIE GOAL: _____

TIME	FOOD	CALORIES	RUNNING TOTAL	HUNGER RATING

TOTAL CALORIC INTAKE: _____

TOTAL CALORIC EXPENDITURE: _____

WATER (8 OZ):

Yay me! _____

_____

_____

Ignite Day 13

THE FOOD LOG　　　　　　DATE: _____ CALORIE GOAL: _____

TIME	FOOD	CALORIES	RUNNING TOTAL	HUNGER RATING

TOTAL CALORIC INTAKE: _____

TOTAL CALORIC EXPENDITURE: _____

WATER (8 OZ):

Yay me! _____

_____

_____

Ignite Day 14

THE FOOD LOG DATE: _____ CALORIE GOAL: _____

TIME	FOOD	CALORIES	RUNNING TOTAL	HUNGER RATING

TOTAL CALORIC INTAKE: _____

TOTAL CALORIC EXPENDITURE: _____

WATER (8 OZ):

Yay me! _____

_____

_____

Ignite Day 15

THE FOOD LOG　　　　　DATE: _____ CALORIE GOAL: _____

TIME	FOOD	CALORIES	RUNNING TOTAL	HUNGER RATING

TOTAL CALORIC INTAKE: _____

TOTAL CALORIC EXPENDITURE: _____

WATER (8 OZ):

Yay me! _____

_____

_____

Ignite Day 16

THE FOOD LOG DATE: _____ CALORIE GOAL: _____

TIME	FOOD	CALORIES	RUNNING TOTAL	HUNGER RATING

TOTAL CALORIC INTAKE: _____

TOTAL CALORIC EXPENDITURE: _____

WATER (8 OZ):

Yay me! _____

_____

_____

THE FOOD LOG   DATE: _____ CALORIE GOAL: _____

TIME	FOOD	CALORIES	RUNNING TOTAL	HUNGER RATING

TOTAL CALORIC INTAKE: _____

TOTAL CALORIC EXPENDITURE: _____

WATER (8 OZ):

Yay me! _____

_____

_____

Ignite Day 18

THE FOOD LOG   DATE: _____ CALORIE GOAL: _____

TIME	FOOD	CALORIES	RUNNING TOTAL	HUNGER RATING

TOTAL CALORIC INTAKE: _____

TOTAL CALORIC EXPENDITURE: _____

WATER (8 OZ):

Yay me! _____

_____

_____

THE FOOD LOG   DATE: _____ CALORIE GOAL: _____

TIME	FOOD	CALORIES	RUNNING TOTAL	HUNGER RATING

TOTAL CALORIC INTAKE: _____

TOTAL CALORIC EXPENDITURE: _____

WATER (8 OZ):

Yay me! _____

_____

_____

Ignite Day 20

DATE: _____ CALORIE GOAL: _____

TIME	FOOD	CALORIES	RUNNING TOTAL	HUNGER RATING

TOTAL CALORIC INTAKE: _____

TOTAL CALORIC EXPENDITURE: _____

WATER (8 OZ):

Yay me! _____

_____

_____

Ignite Day 21

THE FOOD LOG   DATE: _____ CALORIE GOAL: _____

TIME	FOOD	CALORIES	RUNNING TOTAL	HUNGER RATING

TOTAL CALORIC INTAKE: _____

TOTAL CALORIC EXPENDITURE: _____

WATER (8 OZ):

Yay me! _____

_____

_____

Melt Day I

DATE: _____ CALORIE GOAL: _____

TIME	FOOD	CALORIES	RUNNING TOTAL	HUNGER RATING

TOTAL CALORIC INTAKE: _____

TOTAL CALORIC EXPENDITURE: _____

WATER (8 OZ):

Yay me! _____

_____

_____

THE FOOD LOG DATE: _____ CALORIE GOAL: _____

TIME	FOOD	CALORIES	RUNNING TOTAL	HUNGER RATING

TOTAL CALORIC INTAKE: _____

TOTAL CALORIC EXPENDITURE: _____

WATER (8 OZ):

Yay me! _____

_____

_____

Melt Day 3

DATE: _____ CALORIE GOAL: _____

TIME	FOOD	CALORIES	RUNNING TOTAL	HUNGER RATING

TOTAL CALORIC INTAKE: _____

TOTAL CALORIC EXPENDITURE: _____

WATER (8 OZ):

Yay me! _____

_____

_____

THE FOOD LOG DATE: _____ CALORIE GOAL: _____

TIME	FOOD	CALORIES	RUNNING TOTAL	HUNGER RATING

TOTAL CALORIC INTAKE: _____

TOTAL CALORIC EXPENDITURE: _____

WATER (8 OZ):

Yay me! _____

_____

_____

Melt Day 5

THE FOOD LOG DATE: _____ CALORIE GOAL: _____

TIME	FOOD	CALORIES	RUNNING TOTAL	HUNGER RATING

TOTAL CALORIC INTAKE: _____

TOTAL CALORIC EXPENDITURE: _____

WATER (8 OZ): ☐ ☐ ☐ ☐ ☐ ☐ ☐ ☐

Yay me! _____

_____

_____

THE FOOD LOG DATE: _____ CALORIE GOAL: _____

TIME	FOOD	CALORIES	RUNNING TOTAL	HUNGER RATING

TOTAL CALORIC INTAKE: _____

TOTAL CALORIC EXPENDITURE: _____

WATER (8 OZ):

Yay me! _____

_____

_____

Melt Day 7

DATE: _____ CALORIE GOAL: _____

TIME	FOOD	CALORIES	RUNNING TOTAL	HUNGER RATING

TOTAL CALORIC INTAKE: _____

TOTAL CALORIC EXPENDITURE: _____

WATER (8 OZ):

Yay me! _____

_____

_____

THE FOOD LOG　　　DATE: _____ CALORIE GOAL: _____

TIME	FOOD	CALORIES	RUNNING TOTAL	HUNGER RATING

TOTAL CALORIC INTAKE: _____

TOTAL CALORIC EXPENDITURE: _____

WATER (8 OZ):

Yay me! _____

_____

_____

Melt Day 9

DATE: _____ CALORIE GOAL: _____

TIME	FOOD	CALORIES	RUNNING TOTAL	HUNGER RATING

TOTAL CALORIC INTAKE: _____

TOTAL CALORIC EXPENDITURE: _____

WATER (8 OZ): ⬜ ⬜ ⬜ ⬜ ⬜ ⬜ ⬜ ⬜

Yay me! _____

_____

_____

THE FOOD LOG DATE: _____ CALORIE GOAL: _____

TIME	FOOD	CALORIES	RUNNING TOTAL	HUNGER RATING

TOTAL CALORIC INTAKE: _____

TOTAL CALORIC EXPENDITURE: _____

WATER (8 OZ):

Yay me! _____

_____

_____

Melt Day II

THE FOOD LOG DATE: _____ CALORIE GOAL: _____

TIME	FOOD	CALORIES	RUNNING TOTAL	HUNGER RATING

TOTAL CALORIC INTAKE: _____

TOTAL CALORIC EXPENDITURE: _____

WATER (8 OZ): ⬜ ⬜ ⬜ ⬜ ⬜ ⬜ ⬜ ⬜

Yay me! _____

_____

_____

Melt Day 12

THE FOOD LOG   DATE: _____ CALORIE GOAL: _____

TIME	FOOD	CALORIES	RUNNING TOTAL	HUNGER RATING

TOTAL CALORIC INTAKE: _____

TOTAL CALORIC EXPENDITURE: _____

WATER (8 OZ):

Yay me! _____

_____

_____

Melt Day 13

THE FOOD LOG   DATE: _____ CALORIE GOAL: _____

TIME	FOOD	CALORIES	RUNNING TOTAL	HUNGER RATING

TOTAL CALORIC INTAKE: _____

TOTAL CALORIC EXPENDITURE: _____

WATER (8 OZ):

Yay me! _____

_____

_____

Melt Day 14

THE FOOD LOG   DATE: _____ CALORIE GOAL: _____

TIME	FOOD	CALORIES	RUNNING TOTAL	HUNGER RATING

TOTAL CALORIC INTAKE: _____

TOTAL CALORIC EXPENDITURE: _____

WATER (8 OZ):

Yay me! _____

_____

_____

Melt Day 15

DATE: _____ CALORIE GOAL: _____

TIME	FOOD	CALORIES	RUNNING TOTAL	HUNGER RATING

TOTAL CALORIC INTAKE: _____

TOTAL CALORIC EXPENDITURE: _____

WATER (8 OZ):

Yay me! _____

_____

_____

THE FOOD LOG DATE: _____ CALORIE GOAL: _____

TIME	FOOD	CALORIES	RUNNING TOTAL	HUNGER RATING

TOTAL CALORIC INTAKE: _____

TOTAL CALORIC EXPENDITURE: _____

WATER (8 OZ):

Yay me! _____

_____

_____

Melt Day 17

DATE: _____ CALORIE GOAL: _____

TIME	FOOD	CALORIES	RUNNING TOTAL	HUNGER RATING

TOTAL CALORIC INTAKE: _____

TOTAL CALORIC EXPENDITURE: _____

WATER (8 OZ):

Yay me! _____

_____

_____

THE FOOD LOG   DATE: _____ CALORIE GOAL: _____

TIME	FOOD	CALORIES	RUNNING TOTAL	HUNGER RATING

TOTAL CALORIC INTAKE: _____

TOTAL CALORIC EXPENDITURE: _____

WATER (8 OZ):

Yay me! _____

_____

_____

Melt Day 19

DATE: _____ CALORIE GOAL: _____

TIME	FOOD	CALORIES	RUNNING TOTAL	HUNGER RATING

TOTAL CALORIC INTAKE: _____

TOTAL CALORIC EXPENDITURE: _____

WATER (8 OZ):

Yay me! _____

_____

_____

Melt Day 20

THE FOOD LOG   DATE: _____ CALORIE GOAL: _____

TIME	FOOD	CALORIES	RUNNING TOTAL	HUNGER RATING

TOTAL CALORIC INTAKE: _____

TOTAL CALORIC EXPENDITURE: _____

WATER (8 OZ):

Yay me! _____

_____

_____

Melt Day 21

THE FOOD LOG   DATE: _____ CALORIE GOAL: _____

TIME	FOOD	CALORIES	RUNNING TOTAL	HUNGER RATING

TOTAL CALORIC INTAKE: _____

TOTAL CALORIC EXPENDITURE: _____

WATER (8 OZ): ▢ ▢ ▢ ▢ ▢ ▢ ▢ ▢

Yay me! _____

_____

_____

Amy's Favorite Things

Books

Anatomy of the Spirit: The Seven Stages of Power and Healing by Caroline Myss (Aug 26, 1997)

Awaken the Giant Within : How to Take Immediate Control of Your Mental, Emotional, Physical and Financial Destiny! by Anthony Robbins (Nov 1, 1992)

ChiRunning: A Revolutionary Approach to Effortless, Injury-Free Running by Danny Dreyer and Katherine Dreyer (May 5, 2009)

Cook This, Not That! Easy & Awesome 350-Calorie Meals by David Zinczenko and Matt Goulding (Oct 12, 2010)

Leading Women Who Wound: Strategies for Effective Ministry by Sue Edwards and Kelley Mathews (Feb 1, 2009)

Napoleon Hill's Keys to Success: The 17 Principles of Personal Achievement by Napoleon Hill (Oct 1, 1997)

Never Give Up!: Relentless Determination to Overcome Life's Challenges by Joyce Meyer (Nov 17, 2010)

Off the Deep End: The Probably Insane Idea That I Could Swim My Way through a Midlife Crises, and Qualify for the Olympics by W. Hodding Carter (Jun 10, 2008)

The 7 Habits of Highly Effective People: Powerful Lessons in Personal Change by Stephen R. Covey (Nov 9, 2004)

The 5 Love Languages: The Secret to Love That Lasts by Gary Chapman (Jan 1, 2010)

The Seat of the Soul by Gary Zukav (Jan 15, 1990)

The Secret by Rhonda Byrne (Nov 28, 2006)

The Success Principles(TM): How to Get from Where You Are to Where You Want to Be by Jack Canfield and Janet Switzer (Dec 26, 2006)

Your Best Life Now: 7 Steps to Living at |Your Full Potential by Joel Osteen (Aug 20, 2007)

Online Food & Exercise Logs/Tracking

My Fitness Pal: http://www.myfitnesspal.com

Live Strong: http://www.livestrong.com

Recipe Calorie Calculators/Analyzers

Calorie Count: http://caloriecount.about.com/cc/recipe_analysis.php

My Fitness Pal: http://www.myfitnesspal.com/recipe/calculator

Self Nutrition Data: http://nutritiondata.self.com/

Recipe Sites (Free)

Amy Cotta: http://www.amycotta.com

Spark Recipes: http://www.sparkrecipes.com/

Food Network: http://www.foodnetwork
.com/healthy-eating/index.html

Mayo Clinic: http://www.mayoclinic.com/
health/healthy-recipes/RecipeIndex

Prevention Magazine: http://www
.prevention.com/health/cook

Activity/Calorie Burn Calculator

Discovery Health: http://health.discovery
.com/centers/cholesterol/activity/
activity.html

Self Nutrition Data: http://nutritiondata
.self.com/tools/calories-burned

My Fitness Pal: http://www.myfitnesspal
.com/exercise/lookup

Exercise Video Clips

Amy Cotta: http://www.AmyCotta.com

XerciseTV: http://www.youtube.com/
xercisetv

Meal Replacement Shakes, Protein Cookies & Nutritional Products

ViSalus: http://www.
theskinnyjeanschallenge.com

Facebook Pages—Active Living, Giving, and Just for Fun

Six Weeks to Skinny Jeans: http://www
.facebook.com/sixweekstoskinnyjeans

My Fitness Pal: http://www.facebook.com/
myfitnesspal

Team TRI Pink: http://www.facebook.com/
teamtripink

Prevention Magazine: http://www.
facebook.com/preventionmagazine

Iron Girl: http://www.facebook.com/
IronGirlEventSeries

Trek Women: http://www.facebook.com/
TrekWomen

Moms Who Need Wine: http://www
.facebook.com/MomsWhoNeedWine

Amy Cotta: http://www.facebook.com/
authoramycotta

The Boot Campaign: http://www.facebook
.com/bootcampaign

Lone Survivor Foundation: http://www
.facebook.com/lonesurvivorfoundation

Susan G Komen: http://www.facebook.
com/susangkomenforthecure

St Jude Children's Research Hospital:
http://www.facebook.com/stjude

Group Fitness/Super Charge My Skinny!

Zumba: http://www.zumba.com

    Zumba®

    Zumba® Toning

    Zumbatomic® for kids

    Aqua Zumba®

Billy Blanks: http://www.teamtaebo.com/
Tae Bo

Les Mills: http://www.LesMills.com

    BODYCOMBAT

    BODYPUMP

    BODYVIVE

    BODYJAM

    BODYBALANCE/FLOW

    BODYSTEP

    BODYATTACK

    RPM

    SH'BAM

    CX30

Adventure Boot Camp: http://www
.bootcampfinder.com/

Spinning: http://www.spinning.com

Krank Cycle: http://www.krankcycle.com

Indoor Rowing: http://www.concpet2.com

YogaFit: http://www.yogafit.com/

Balanced Body Pilates: http://www
.pilates.com/BBAPP/V/community/
studio-finder.html

Non-group Fitness or Gym Related/ Super Charge My Skinny!

U.S. Master Swimming: http://www.usms
.org/

Hiking Trails: http://www.trails.com/

Mountain bike Trails: http://www
.singletracks.com/mountainbike/

trails.php?gclid=CPaR
_czJ26oCFQwr7Aod-3b16w

Runs / running routes: http://www
.mapmyrun.com/

Cycling routes: http://www.mapmyride.com/

USA Triathlon: www.usatriathlon.org

Fitness Equipment & Accessories

Amy Cotta: http://www.AmyCotta.com

Fun, Functional Fashions

PUMA: http://www.shop.puma.com

Reebok: www.reebok.com/Shop

Athleta: http://athleta.gap.com/

Lu Lu Lemon: www.lululemon.com

Become a Rock Star!

Skinny Jeans Challenge

☐ Take before photos and measurements. (See page 67.)

☐ Join the community at www.amycotta.com & Facebook.com/
SixWeeksToSkinnyJeans.

☐ Join www.myfitnesspal.com and start tracking your daily food & exercise.

☐ Invite friends to join the challenge with you. (See Can-Do Society on page 26.)

☐ Follow the program like it's your new religion.

☐ Frequently post updates on your Facebook page, Twitter, amycotta.com and
Facebook: Six Weeks to Skinny Jeans.

☐ Share your results and before and after photos on www.amycotta.com to be
eligible to win prizes!

Your Skinny Jeans Are Waiting!

Notes

Chapter 2

1. Kirsti A. Dyer, "How to Eat Healthy on a Budget," *Suite101*, published October 25, 2009, www.suite101.com/content/how-to-eat-healthy-on-a-budget-a94854.

Chapter 3

1. Selene Yeager, "Rev Your Metabolism: Drink Water," *Prevention*, last updated January 3, 2006, www.prevention.com/health/weight-loss/success-stories/water-and-weight-loss/article/211388dc78803110VgnVCM10000013281eac_____/.
2. NutriBase 9 Professional Nutrition and Fitness Software, accessed December 12, 2010, www.nutribase.com/foodterm.shtml.
3. "Eat Any Sugar Alcohol Lately?" Yale–New Haven Hospital, accessed December 12, 2010, www.ynhh.org/about-us/sugar_alcohol.aspx.
4. Katherine Zeratsky, R.D., Nutrition and Healthy Eating Q&A, Mayo Clinic, accessed December 12, 2010, www.mayoclinic.com/health/multigrain/AN02047.
5. Julie Knapp, "17 Eco-Food Labels Decoded," Mother Nature Network, published April 26, 2010, www.mnn.com/food/healthy-eating-recipes/stories/17-eco-food-labels-decoded.

Chapter 4

1. Macaroni Grill's nutrition information can be found at www.macaronigrill.com.
2. Livestrong.com, "Facts on Colon Cleanse Benefits," last updated on November 18, 2009, www.livestrong.com/article/2810.

Chapter 8

1. Nutrition information for many restaurants can be found at their Web sites. Subway and Wendy's information came from www.subway.com and www.wendys.com, respectively.

Chapter 9

1. Panda Express nutrition information can be found at www.pandaexpress.com. I have nothing against Panda Express. As I said, the goal of restaurants is to make their foods taste good, not to keep you skinny.
2. Shirley Archer, "More Good Reasons for Athletes to Do Yoga," *Idea Fitness Journal* 2, no. 3 (March 2005), www.ideafit.com/fitness-library/more-good-reasons-athletes-do-yoga.

Chapter 10

1. Amanda Gardner, "Cutting TV Time Burns More Calories," *U.S. News & World Report,* accessed December 22, 2010, http://health.usnews.com/health-news/diet-fitness/fitness/articles/2009/12/14/cutting-tv-time-burns-more-calories.html.

2. Jack Canfield, *The Success Principles: How to Get from Where You Are to Where You Want to Be* (New York: Harper, 2006).

3. Ibid.

Chapter 11

1. Permission to reprint has been granted by the copyright owner, IDEA Health & Fitness Association, www.ideafit.com. Reproduction to reprint without permission is strictly prohibited. All rights reserved.

2. "Alcohol and Calories: Does Drinking Cause Weight Gain?" Elle.com blog, *Shine,* published February 25, 2010, http://shine.yahoo.com/channel/health/alcohol-and-calories-does-drinking-cause-weight-gain-878173/.

Index

Boldface page references indicate photographs. Underscored references indicate boxed text.